Moorfields Eye Hospital

230

UNS

WITHDRAWN

GW00693991

**Joint Library of Ophthalmology, Moorfields
Eye Hospital & UCL Institute of Ophthalmology**

Library website: www.ucl.ac.uk/library/iophth
Tel: 020 7608 6814 / 020 7566 2084

To be returned on or before the date marked below

To renew your loans online, you need to go to the library
catalogue http://library.ucl.ac.uk and log into My Account
with your barcode number starting 028 and your 4 digit PIN

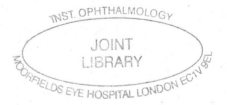
INST. OPHTHALMOLOGY
JOINT
LIBRARY
MOORFIELDS EYE HOSPITAL LONDON EC1V 9EL

WITHDRAWN

INST OPHTHALMOLOGY

JOINT
LIBRARY

MOORFIELDS EYE HOSPITAL LONDON EC1V

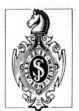

Renate Unsöld   Wolfgang Seeger

Compressive
Optic Nerve Lesions
at the Optic Canal

Pathogenesis – Diagnosis – Treatment

Collaborators
M. Bach H.-R. Eggert G. Greeven J. DeGroot

With 88 Figures in 180 Separate Illustrations
Partly in Color

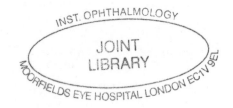

INST. OPHTHALMOLOGY
JOINT LIBRARY
MOORFIELDS EYE HOSPITAL LONDON EC1V 9EL

Springer-Verlag
Berlin Heidelberg NewYork
London Paris Tokyo

Cover photo:
Axial anatomic section through
the intracranial optic canal (Fig. 6)

This work is subject to copyright. All rights are reserved, whether the whole or part of the
material is concerned, specifically the rights of translation, reprinting, re-use of illustrations,
recitation, broadcasting, reproduction on microfilms or in other ways, and storage in data
banks. Duplication of this publication or parts thereof is only permitted under the provisions
of the German Copyright Law of September 9, 1965, in its version of June 24, 1985, and a
copyright fee must always be paid. Violations fall under the prosecution act of the German
Copyright Law.

© Springer-Verlag Berlin Heidelberg 1989

The use of registered names, trademarks, etc. in this publication does not imply, even in the
absence of a specific statement, that such names are exempt from the relevant protective laws
and regulations and therefore free for general use.

Product liability: The publisher can give no guarantee for information about drug dosage and
application thereof contained in this book. In every individual case the respective user must
check its accuracy by consulting other pharmaceutical literature.

Reproduction of the figures: Gustav Dreher GmbH, Stuttgart

2121/3130-543210 – Printed on acid-free paper

ISBN-13:978-3-642-73384-0   e-ISBN-13:978-3-642-73382-6
DOI: 10.1007/978-3-642-73382-6

William Fletcher Hoyt
In Honor of His 60th Birthday

Authors

RENATE UNSÖLD, Prof. Dr. med., Universitätsaugenklinik,
Moorenstraße 5, D-4000 Düsseldorf

WOLFGANG SEEGER, Prof. Dr. med., Direktor der Neurochirurgischen
Universitätsklinik, Hugstetter Straße 55, D-7800 Freiburg

MICHAEL BACH, Dr. rer. nat., Universitätsaugenklinik,
Killianstraße 5, D-7800 Freiburg

HANS-RUDOLF EGGERT, Priv.-Doz. Dr. med., Neurochirurgische Universitätsklinik,
Hugstetter Straße 55, D-7800 Freiburg

GABRIELE GREEVEN, Dr. med., Chefärztin der Radiologischen Abteilung,
St. Elisabeth-Krankenhaus, D-5450 Neuwied

JACK DE GROOT, MD, PhD, Professor, Department of Anatomy,
University of California Medical School, Parnassus Avenue,
San Francisco, CA 94143, USA

Contents

1
Introduction

The optic canal, in particular its intracranial end, represents a "locus minoris resistentiae" for optic nerve compression in a variety of pathologic conditions. The intracranial optic nerve shares the limited space within this narrow passage with the carotid and ophthalmic artery, all being surrounded by bone and rigid dura. Any pathological condition going along with an increase of soft tissue volume, such as in optic nerve sheath tumors, parasellar neoplasms, dolichoectasia of the carotid and/ or ophthalmic artery, hematomas, etc., or reduction of the lumen of the bony optic canal by hyperpneumatization of the sphenoid sinus, hyperostosis or developmental abnormalities must act as a space-occupying lesion causing optic nerve compression either by pressing the nerve against the vessel or the neighboring dura or bone.

The spectrum of clinical signs and symptoms of optic nerve compression in this area is rather wide and includes acute as well as slowly progressive visual loss and all kinds of visual field defects in the presence of a normal disk, papilledema, primary optic atrophy or cavernous optic atrophy mimicking various clinical disease entities such as retrobulbar optic neuritis, anterior and posterior ischemic optic neuropathy, soft glaucoma and others. Some of the lesions causing optic nerve compression in this area are rather small and need to be visualized or excluded by thin section CT such as pneumosinus dilatans of the sphenoid bone, dolichoectasia of the internal carotid artery, small meningiomas around the optic foramen and others. Early diagnosis is however necessary, since further development of refined microsurgical techniques and new approaches have considerably reduced the rate of mortality and morbidity in the neurosurgical treatment of compressive optic nerve lesions. Adequate surgical treatment has been proven to allow not only consolidation but also improvement of visual function when the diagnosis is established in time, i.e., *before* significant optic atrophy has occurred.

This publication aims to draw attention to this predilected anatomic area for optic nerve compression by a variety of lesions and particularly to resurrect the concept of dolichoectatic internal carotid and ophthalmic arteries and hyperpneumatizations (pneumosinus dilatans) being instrumental in compressing the optic nerve within the area of the optic canal.

The literature of these lesions is reviewed, the clinical signs and symptoms, the radiologic findings, the techniques of neurosurgical therapy and the surgical results are described on the basis of our own cases. The clinical implications and therapeutic conclusions are discussed.

2

A Narrow Passage – Anatomic Considerations

Topography of the Optic Canal Representing a Predilection of Nerve Compression with Various Pathologic Conditions

R. Unsöld, W. Seeger, J. De Groot

At the intracranial end of the optic foramen in higher primates and human beings, the internal carotid and ophthalmic artery share a narrow space surrounded by bones or rigid dural structures.

There, the optic nerve overlies the internal carotid artery immediately beneath the dural fold overcrossing the opening of the inner end of the optic canal between the limbus sphenoidalis and the anterior clinoid process representing a rigid fibrous connective cord. Medially this space is limited by the sphenoid sinus and the lesser wing of the sphenoid bone, laterally by the anterior clinoid process and inferiorly by the floor of the optic foramen and the dura covering the cavernous sinus. Just within this narrow passage the carotid artery gives rise to the ophthalmic artery which follows the optic nerve at its inferior surface through the optic canal within its dural sheath.

Whereas in lower animals the internal carotid arteries are rather small vessels of minor importance, in higher primates they become – due to the overdimensional development of the cerebral cortex – rather large, thus reducing the space between the intracranial optic nerve and the overlying dural fold covering the intracranial optic canal. Particularly in human beings, considerable extension of life expectancy into a seventh, eighth or ninth decade may go along with significant arteriosclerotic vascular changes causing weakening of the elastic elements of the vessel wall followed by ectasia and elongation of the arteries ("dolichoectasia") and secondary changes of the vessel wall mainly responsible for the increase of the vascular diameter. With age, particularly in hypertensive and diabetic individuals or patients with other vascular diseases, the increased volume of the internal carotid and/or ophthalmic artery may act as a space-occupying lesion within this narrow passage in which these vessels cannot expand other than in an anterior and superior direction into the intracranial opening of the optic canal and towards the dural fold, resulting in optic nerve compression and therefore the threat of blindness.

But also any other lesion causing an increased volume of soft tissue or narrowing of this space, for instance due to increased pneumatisation of the sphenoid bone, hyperostosis or developmental bony anomalies, may cause nerve compression either against the carotid and ophthalmic artery or the surrounding bony and dural structures.

In dolichoectasia and saccular aneurysms of the carotid artery, the vessel usually pushes the nerve medially and upward against the dural fold, as has been impressively demonstrated by autoptic findings (Fig. 13) causing a deep impression and focal demyelination within the underlying nerve, as well as compression of the superficial vessels supplying the nerve. Supratentorial tumors, brain edema and hematomas may displace the nerve downward, pressing it against the internal carotid artery and the inferior portion of the bony optic canal. Suprasellar tumors, aneurysms, or abnormal vascular loops may lead to a distention and distortion of the nerve, which may become pressed against any neighboring structure, resulting in focal optic nerve damage causing a variety of visual field defects, as clinically observed in numerous patients in which the findings could be verified during surgery, autopsy, or both.

There are certain anatomical peculiarities representing predisposing factors for optic nerve compression in the area of the optic foramen, which need to be taken into account in individual cases:

1. The degree of pneumatization of the sphenoid sinus and lesser wing of the sphenoid bone. (Luxury or excessive pneumatization of the sphenoid sinus particularly of the anterior clinoid process usually continuing from the sphenoid sinus or a posterior ethmoid air cell may reduce the lumen of the bony optic canal by itself acting as a space-occupying lesion or, when dolichoectatic changes of the internal carotid artery occur, may increase the danger of optic nerve compression.)

2. The position of the chiasm determining the length of the intracranial optic nerve and therefore its flexibility, allowing for some escape from space-occupying lesions in this area. (Patients with a prefixed chiasm show less flexibility of the optic nerve and therefore tend to develop earlier optic nerve compression in the presence of a soft tissue volume increase than patients with a postfixed chiasm.)

In patients with luxury pneumatization of the sphenoid sinus and lesser wing of the sphenoid bone with a prefixed chiasm, even slight dolichoectasia of the internal carotid artery may lead to optic nerve compression, whereas in patients with moderate pneumatization and a postfixed chiasm the more flexible optic nerve may tolerate a considerably greater amount of dolichoectasia or soft tissue volume increase by mass lesions, before optic nerve compression occurs. Recognition of these anatomical details is an indispensable precondition for reliable neuroradiological assessment in patients with possible optic nerve compression in the region of the optic canal.

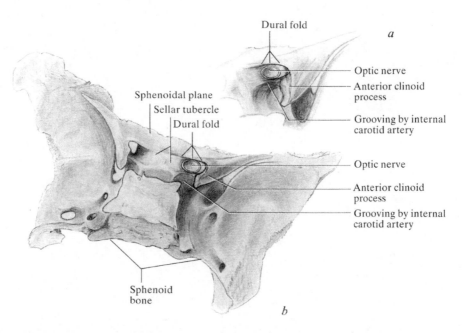

Fig. 1. (*a*) Drawing of the sphenoid bone viewed from above, laterally and behind. The internal carotid artery causes deep grooving into the bone along its intracavernous portion and beneath the intracranial end of the optic canal. (*b*) Slightly magnified view of the intracranial opening of the optic canal as viewed from behind. The bony groove of the internal carotid artery forms the floor of the optic canal. In individuals with arteriosclerotic dolichoectasia of the artery the ectatic and elongated vessel may groove itself deeper and forward into the optic canal, which may become eroded. Note the sharp dural fold overcrossing the intracranial end of the optic canal

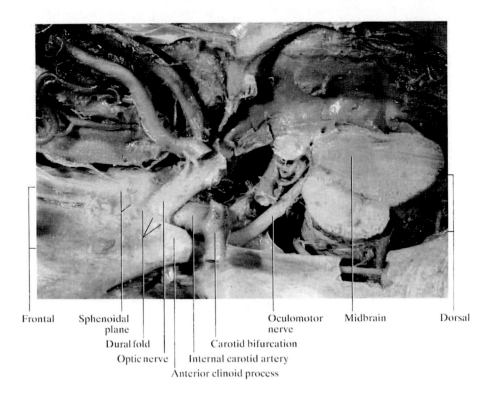

Frontal   Sphenoidal   Oculomotor   Midbrain   Dorsal
           plane   nerve
           Dural fold   Carotid bifurcation
           Optic nerve   Internal carotid artery
                 Anterior clinoid process

Fig. 2. Anatomic dissection of the anterior skull base, viewed from above and laterally. The slightly enlarged internal carotid artery elevates the optic nerve, pressing it against the dural fold forming the roof of the intracranial opening of the optic canal

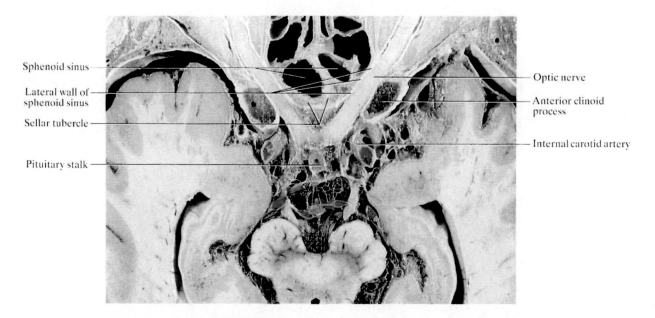

Sphenoid sinus

Lateral wall of sphenoid sinus

Sellar tubercle

Pituitary stalk

Optic nerve

Anterior clinoid process

Internal carotid artery

Fig. 3. Axial anatomic section through the optic canal in the optimal plane for optic nerve evaluation (-10 to $-15°$ to the orbitomeatal base line). Note the topographic relationship of the lateral wall of the sphenoid sinus, the optic nerve, the internal artery, and anterior clinoid process at the intracranial opening of the optic canal. The internal carotid artery is of normal caliber

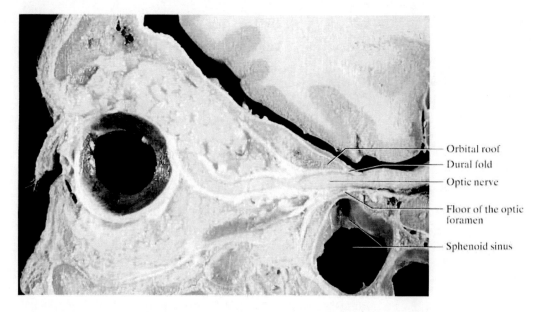

Orbital roof

Dural fold

Optic nerve

Floor of the optic foramen

Sphenoid sinus

Fig. 4. Anatomic section parallel to the course of the optic canal. The bony roof of the optic canal is shorter than its floor. The intracranial opening is formed by a dural fold. The course and diameter of the optic canal depends considerably on the degree of pneumatization of the sphenoid sinus, which is minor in the dissected individual

7

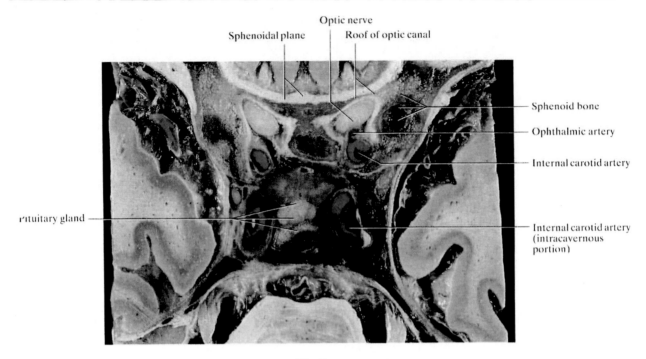

Sphenoidal plane

Optic nerve

Roof of optic canal

Sphenoid bone

Ophthalmic artery

Internal carotid artery

Pituitary gland

Internal carotid artery
(intracavernous
portion)

Fig. 5

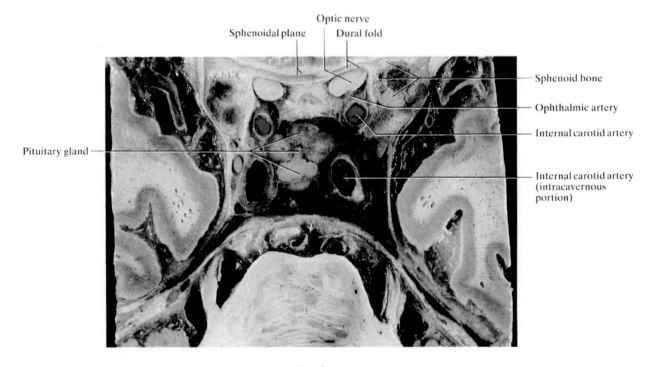

Sphenoidal plane

Optic nerve

Dural fold

Sphenoid bone

Ophthalmic artery

Internal carotid artery

Pituitary gland

Internal carotid artery
(intracavernous
portion)

Fig. 6

Figs. 5, 6. Axial anatomic sections through the anterior skull base at the level of the intraorbital (Fig. 5) and intracranial (Fig. 6) opening of the optic foramen. The narrow space shared by the optic nerve and the underlying internal carotid artery is surrounded by bone and dura. Note the ophthalmic artery arising from the internal carotid artery within this narrow passage

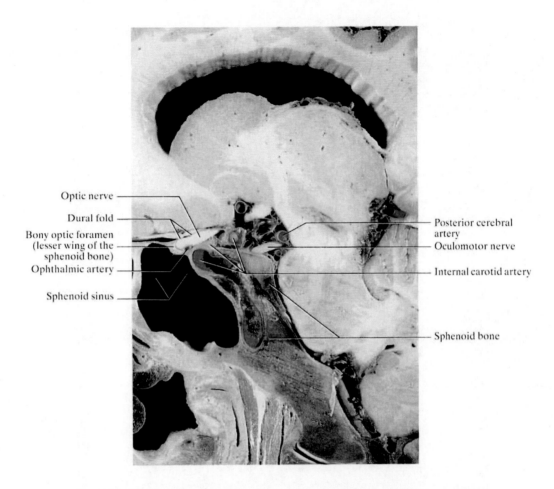

Optic nerve

Dural fold

Bony optic foramen
(lesser wing of the
sphenoid bone)

Ophthalmic artery

Sphenoid sinus

Posterior cerebral
artery

Oculomotor nerve

Internal carotid artery

Sphenoid bone

Fig. 7. Parasagittal anatomic section through the intracranial optic nerve and canal. Note the optic nerve directly overlying the vessel wall beneath the dural fold. Configuration and space of this passage depends considerably on the degree of pneumatization. Note also the section of the ophthalmic artery arising just at the convexity of the carotid siphon. The carotid artery has caused deep grooving in the bony wall of the well-pneumatized sphenoid sinus

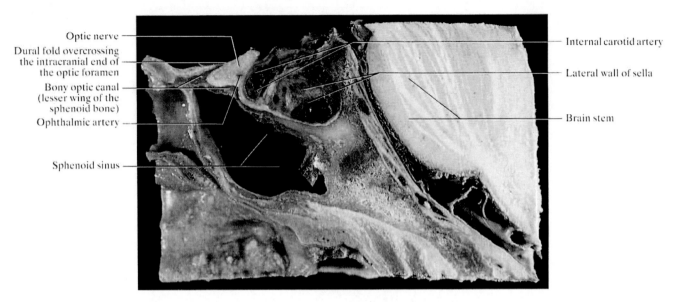

Optic nerve

Dural fold overcrossing the intracranial end of the optic foramen

Bony optic canal (lesser wing of the sphenoid bone)

Ophthalmic artery

Sphenoid sinus

Internal carotid artery

Lateral wall of sella

Brain stem

Fig. 8

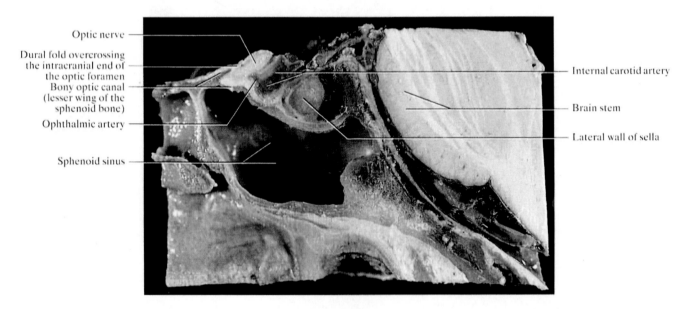

Optic nerve

Dural fold overcrossing the intracranial end of the optic foramen

Bony optic canal (lesser wing of the sphenoid bone)

Ophthalmic artery

Sphenoid sinus

Internal carotid artery

Brain stem

Lateral wall of sella

Fig. 9

Figs. 8–11. Sequential parasagittal anatomic sections at 1 mm distance from the lateral to the medial portion of the optic foramen. Note close contact of nerve and vessel through all sections. The space is limited by the dural fold overcrossing the inner end of the optic foramen and the configuration of the lateral wall of the sphenoid sinus depending on the degree of pneumatization and the caliber of the internal carotid artery

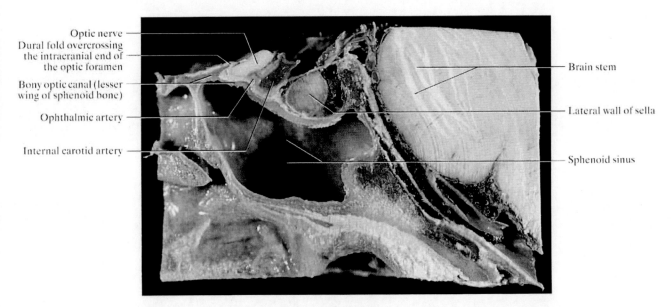

Optic nerve

Dural fold overcrossing the intracranial end of the optic foramen

Bony optic canal (lesser wing of sphenoid bone)

Ophthalmic artery

Internal carotid artery

Brain stem

Lateral wall of sella

Sphenoid sinus

Fig. 10

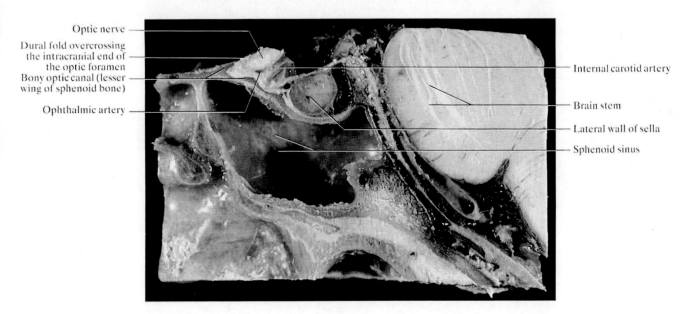

Optic nerve

Dural fold overcrossing the intracranial end of the optic foramen

Bony optic canal (lesser wing of sphenoid bone)

Ophthalmic artery

Internal carotid artery

Brain stem

Lateral wall of sella

Sphenoid sinus

Fig. 11

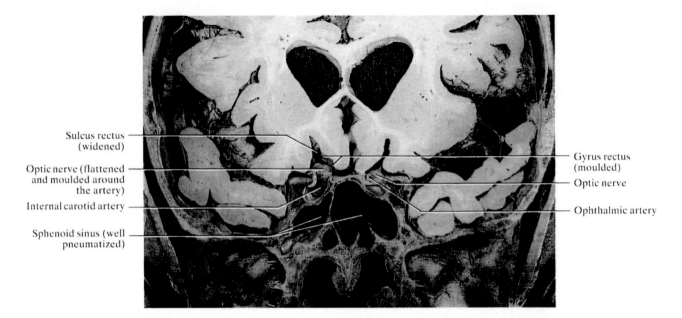

Sulcus rectus (widened)

Optic nerve (flattened and moulded around the artery)

Internal carotid artery

Sphenoid sinus (well pneumatized)

Gyrus rectus (moulded)

Optic nerve

Ophthalmic artery

Fig. 12. Coronal anatomic section through the intracranial end of the optic foramen in an individual with dolichoectatic internal carotid arteries and luxury pneumatization of the sphenoid sinus. The right optic nerve is crossly elevated, flattened and molded around the artery and has caused widening of the overlying sulcus and molding of the neighboring gyrus rectus

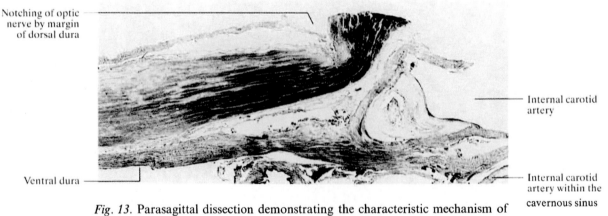

Notching of optic nerve by margin of dorsal dura

Internal carotid artery

Ventral dura

Internal carotid artery within the cavernous sinus

Fig. 13. Parasagittal dissection demonstrating the characteristic mechanism of optic nerve compression by a dolichoectatic carotid artery at the intracranial opening of the optic foramen. "An enlarged sclerotic carotid artery presses the nerve against the margin of the dorsal dural duplication and produces a deep notching of the nerve associated with demyelination and atrophy of dorsal fibers. Part of the artery is located within the cavernous sinus (tangential cut)." Courtesy of Dr. Lindenberg. (From: Lindenberg et al. 1973)

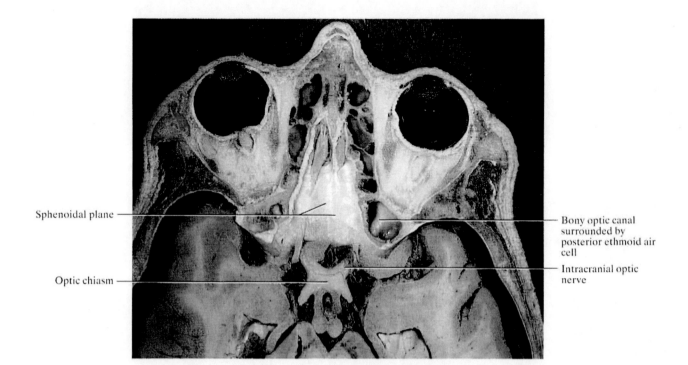

Sphenoidal plane

Optic chiasm

Bony optic canal
surrounded by
posterior ethmoid air
cell

Intracranial optic
nerve

Fig. 14. Axial anatomic section at the level of the chiasm showing an anatomical variation. The optic canals are surrounded by hyperpneumatized ethmoid air cells. When hyperpneumatization causes bone erosion pneumosinus dilatans may result in optic nerve compression. Ethmoid surgery may become dangerous for visual function

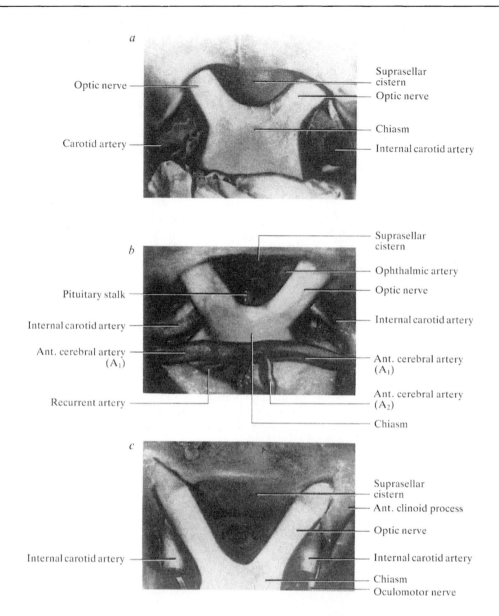

_a_

Optic nerve ——————————

Carotid artery ——————————

Suprasellar
cistern ——————————
Optic nerve ——————————

Chiasm ——————————

Internal carotid artery ——————————

_b_

Pituitary stalk ——————————

Internal carotid artery ——————————

Ant. cerebral artery
(A₁) ——————————

Recurrent artery ——————————

Suprasellar
cistern ——————————

Ophthalmic artery ——————————

Optic nerve ——————————

Internal carotid artery ——————————

Ant. cerebral artery
(A₁) ——————————

Ant. cerebral artery
(A₂) ——————————

Chiasm ——————————

_c_

Internal carotid artery ——————————

Suprasellar
cistern ——————————

Ant. clinoid process ——————————

Optic nerve ——————————

Internal carotid artery ——————————

Chiasm ——————————
Oculomotor nerve ——————————

Fig. 15 a–c. Schematic drawing demonstrating the position of the chiasm related to the intracranial opening of the optic canal. (_a_) Prefixed chiasm; the chiasm is situated close to the intracranial opening of the optic canals allowing less flexibility of the nerve in the case of compression from below or above. (_b_) Normal position of chiasm. (_c_) Postfixed chiasm. The chiasm lies far posterior and superior, the intracranial portion of the optic nerves is of considerable length and allows more flexibility in the case of compression from below or above. (After Miller 1982, p. 61)

3
The Clinical Signs and Symptoms
of Optic Nerve Compression and Clinical Disease Entities
Masking Compressive Lesions

3.1
Ophthalmoscopic Findings. Visual Loss, Visual Field Defects, Afferent Pupillary Defect, Color Vision

R. Unsöld

The clinical signs and symptoms of surgically and autoptically proven lesions in the region of the optic canal vary considerably and may mimic any other suprasellar compressive lesion. The most frequent complaint is visual loss, which may be insidious, occasionally intermittent or rather acute. Slowly progressive visual loss is thought to be characteristic for slowly expanding or growing lesions, such as for instance meningeomas or pneumosinus dilatans, but it has also been observed in vascular lesions such as dolichoectasia or saccular aneurysms of the internal carotid artery (Michel 1877; Schloffer 1934; Mitts and McQueen 1965; Walsh and Hoyt 1969; Walsh 1971; Kennerdell and Maroon 1976; Hollenhorst et al. 1978; Wilson 1981; Miller 1982; Hirst et al. 1982, and others). On the other hand, meningeomas and pneumosinus dilatans may also cause intermittent, subacute or even acute visual loss (Torma and Koskinen 1961; Susac 1977; Wright 1980; Wilson 1981, and others). Acute visual loss is usually thought to represent a "vascular event", and when it occurs with slowly growing or expanding lesions it is thought to represent a sign of hemorrhage into a pre-existing tumor, acute necrosis and edema, for instance in pituitary apoplexy, or a sign of compression of parts of the vascular supply, when the pressure reaches a critical level. In all cases immediate surgical decompression may restore at least part of the function.

At the onset of visual loss there may already be optic atrophy (Behr 1910; Schloffer 1934; Mitts and McQueen 1965; Walsh 1971; Lisch 1976; Wright et al. 1980; Wilson 1981; Miller 1982, and others), occasionally with cupping of the optic disk in the presence of low intraocular pressure (Thiel 1930; McQueen and

Ray 1947; Trobe et al. 1980; Miller 1982; Kupersmith and Krohn 1984), whereas in other patients with neoplastic or vascular lesions at the optic canal a normal optic disk or various degrees of papilledema have been encountered (Michel 1977; Behr 1910; Alpers and Wolman 1931; Caramazza 1932; Schloffer 1934; Yaskin and Schlezinger 1934; Pfingst 1936; Marchesani 1937; Glees 1938; Tassman 1944; Parin 1951; Mitts and McQueen 1965; Walsh and Hoyt 1969; Kennerdell and Maroon 1975; Tomsak et al. 1980; Miller 1982, and others). One of the autoptically proven cases of optic nerve compression by a dolecholectatic artery showed besides papilledema the characteristic nerve fiber changes as seen in "neuroretinitis" (Alpers and Wolman 1931). Particularly in cases with dolecholectatic internal carotid arteries one frequently finds optic atrophy already in the other eye, when acute visual loss occurs with the ophthalmoscopic picture of papilledema reminiscent of the "Foster Kennedy Syndrome".

It remains totally unresolved why the same kind of lesion in some patients causes papilledema, whereas it leads to primary optic atrophy in others. Differences in the mechanism of local compression may possibly play a role and are also probably reflected by the different types of visual field defects encountered in patients with lesions around the optic foramen. One could imagine that diffuse optic nerve compression within the canal might primarily compromise axonal transport mechanisms leading to papilledema, whereas more local compression, for instance by the dural fold, the artery or the anterior clinoid process, may lead to pressure occlusion of smaller supplying vessels, eventually resulting in focal ischemia and atrophy. Absolute scotomas in certain areas of the visual field in patients who underwent decompression and afterwards regained immediate and almost complete restoration of vision may indicate such a vascular compressive mechanism. Actually one encounters all kinds of visual field defects in surgically and autoptically proven lesions of this area. Visual loss usually due to a central or centrocoecal scotoma is frequently observed in neoplastic and vascular compressive lesions as well as after trauma to the optic canal (Caramazza 1932; Schloffer 1934; Yaskin and Schlezinger 1942; McLean and Ray 1947; Ricci and Werner 1957; Harms 1963; Schlezinger and Thompson 1967; Sugita et al. 1975; Hollenhorst et al. 1978; Wilson 1981; Gutman 1984, and others). But all other types of visual field defects with and without central scotomas have been described in the presence of compressive lesions particularly at the intracranial opening of the optic canal such as *concentric restriction* (Behr 1910; Schloffer 1934; Yaskin and Schlezinger

1942; Walsh 1971; Hollenhorst et al. 1978; Wilson 1981, and others), *altitudinal defects* (Sandford et al. 1936; McLean and Ray 1947; Walsh and Hoyt 1969; Lisch 1976; Enoksson and Johansson 1973; Hollenhorst et al. 1978; Kupersmith and Krohn 1984; Spoor et al. 1986, and others), *arcuate defects* (Caramazza 1932; McLean and Ray 1947; Ricci and Werner 1957; Kearns and Rucker 1958, and others), as well as *temporal* (Ricci and Werner 1957; Bergaust 1963; Trobe et al. 1974; Matsuo et al. 1980, and others), and *nasal scotomas* (Caramazza 1932; Yaskin and Schlezinger 1942; O'Connell and Du Boulay 1973; Kupersmith and Krohn 1984, and others), and *any combination of visual field defects* (McLean and Ray 1947; Harms 1958; Walsh and Gass 1960; Mills and McQueen 1965; Schmidt and Bührman 1977; Wilson 1981, and others).

Sometimes a *central scotoma* is followed by an altitudinal defect as compression increases (McLean and Ray 1947). The mechanism of tumors or dolichoectatic vessels pressing the nerve upward against the dural fold overlying the intracranial end of the optic foramen has been well documented in surgically and autoptically proven cases frequently causing *central scotomas and* altitudinal, mostly *inferior visual field defects* (Bernheimer 1891; Otto 1902; Wilbrand and Sänger 1913; Fuchs 1922; Schloffer 1934; Lindenberg et al. 1973; Schmidt and Bührman 1977, and others). Total compression of the lateral portion of the optic nerve by a dolichoectatic internal carotid artery resulting in local atrophy and thinning of the nerve has been well documented by Sacks and Lindenberg 1969; Lindenberg et al. 1973, and others. This kind of focal compression seems to be the morphologic substrate of nasal and binasal visual field defects described in arteriosclerotic patients with dolichoectatic arteries. Optic nerve compression against the carotid artery or the bony optic canal from above in the presence of space-occupying supratentorial lesions may explain isolated superior altitudinal defects (Schmidt and Bührman 1977, and others). Displacement and distortion of the optic nerve in neoplastic or vascular lesions may lead to the differences of local compression reflected by the variety of visual field defects. Apparent disproportion for instance of the degree of dolichoectasia of the internal carotid artery and the degree of visual loss and visual field defects may be due to anatomic pecularities in individual cases such as the previously mentioned hyperpneumatization of the sphenoid sinus and lesser wing of the sphenoid bone or a prefixed chiasm, the former reducing the lumen of the optic canal and the latter reducing the flexibility of the nerve and its chance to escape from the compressing artery.

In unilateral lesions, the proof of an afferent pupillary defect with the swinging-flashlight test in the absence of an intraocular explanation serves as an objective and reliable sign of optic nerve damage and requires exclusion of a compressive mechanism. The test should be carried out in a dark room in order to produce wide pupils and therefore a large amplitude of pupillary constriction; illumination should be diffuse, achieved by illuminating both eyes from below, and the light source should be swung at a time interval of 3–5 seconds. In the presence of a pupillary defect, on swinging the flashlight from the unaffected eye to the affected eye one will see pupillary dilation, or at least less initial constriction. Loss of color perception or color desaturation is another important clinical symptom indicating optic nerve compression, particularly if it develops during the disease process. Careful evaluation of the visual evoked potentials may give further confirmation of the compressive mechanism. The problems of interpretation of the VEP are described in detail in the following section.

To summarize, optic nerve compression should be suspected or excluded in any case of visual loss and with any type of visual field defect that cannot be explained by ophthalmoscopically visible intraocular lesions. The presence of optic atrophy with and without cupping of the disk or papilledema is an important additional indication for neuroradiological examination, but an optic disk of normal appearance does not exclude nerve compression at an early stage of the disease. The proof of an afferent pupillary defect or desaturation or loss of previously existent color perception are further important indicators of a compressive lesion.

The clinical signs and symptoms of optic nerve compression frequently mimic certain clinical disease entities, the erroneous diagnosis of which may delay timely diagnosis and treatment of the compressive lesion.

The most frequent disease entity masking a compressive mechanism is "optic neuritis" in patients with central scotomas which show some degree of improvement due to the intermittent character of the compression, as has been well described in tumors and vascular lesions such as dolichoectatic vessels and or aneurysms. Any case of "optic neuritis" which is not characterized by the typical course with pain during eye movements in the initial stage, early improvement within about 3 weeks with resolution of the central scotoma and the sign of increased latency in the VEP of the other eye requires neuroradiological investigation. The latter is also indicated in patients with optic disk cupping in the presence of normal intraocular pressure.

Suprasellar mass lesions as well as compression by dolichoectatic vessels have been proven to cause this type of optic atrophy, which is difficult to distinguish from glaucomatous cupping (Thiel 1930; McLean and Ray 1947; Trobe et al. 1980; Kupersmith and Krohn 1984). We have observed a rather high frequency of severe dolichoectatic changes of the internal carotid artery in this group of patients as compared with other patients in the same age group and with the same underlying systemic diseases. Possibly chronic optic nerve compression by dolichoectatic vessels may lead to congestion of the axoplasmatic transport and axonal damage at the lamina cribrosa even with normal intraocular pressure. Presence of papilledema in a considerable number of patients with a surgically or autoptically proven compressive mechanism in the area of the optic foramen probably due to disturbances of axoplasmic transport could be taken as evidence for the existence of such a mechanism (McLead 1980; Miller 1982).

Another clinical disease entity that, despite numerous publications, remains rather poorly understood is that of anterior and posterior ischemic optic neuropathy. Although this entity has been thought to result from ciliary artery occlusion, and similar pathological changes could experimentally be shown to occur after ligation of these arteries in monkeys, other investigators could not reliably reproduce these experiments (Anderson et al. 1974). Some authors believe that optic disk swelling in anterior ischemic optic neuropathy is due to disturbances of axoplasmic flow (McLeod et al. 1980). The population of patients with "anterior and posterior ischemic optic neuropathy (non-arteritic group)" shares some prominent clinical features with the population suffering from surgically and autoptically proven optic nerve compression by dolichoectatic carotid arteries: 1. Sudden onset of visual loss; 2. papilledema; 3. the type of visual field defect (in patients with anterior ischemic optic neuropathy 46% show inferior altitudinal defects, 16% partial inferior defects, and about 20% central scotomas, altogether 82% of the patients have the typical visual defects observed in patients with proven compression by a dolichoectatic internal carotid artery); 4. predilection for this disease in hypertensive and diabetic patients (Bogen and Glaser 1975; Hayreh 1979; Ellenberger 1979; Miller 1982; Repka et al. 1983; Quiggly et al. 1985).

Another very interesting finding in three patients with anterior ischemic optic neuropathy who underwent postmortem quantification of the remaining optic nerve fibers showed that in all three patients with non-arteriitic ischemic optic neuropathy

19

there was complete loss of the superior half of each nerve and loss of the peripheral fibers in the other half in the absence of specific small vessel occlusion. This finding could well be explained by the mechanism of optic nerve compression by a dolichoectatic internal carotid artery against the dural fold above the intracranial end of the optic canal as demonstrated in a rather large number of surgically and autoptically proven cases of dolichoectasia and in one case of pneumosinus dilatans (Case 6). The presence of diffuse neuronal damage in the other lower half of the nerve seems easier to explain by a compressive mechanism than by affection of another ciliary artery, which would be more likely to result in total axonal loss. In about 10% of the cases with anterior ischemic optic neuropathy one observes cavernous optic atrophy (cupping of the optic disk) as has also been observed in proven compressive lesions. Finally, the association of "vascular" third nerve palsy and anterior ischemic optic neuropathy could also be interpreted as a sign of nerve compression due to dolichoectatic changes of the internal carotid artery (Bogousslavsky and Steck 1986). We have frequently observed massive dolichoectatic changes of the intracavernous portion of the carotid artery in patients with "vascular third nerve palsies" with spontaneous recovery in the absence of compressive mass lesions. Particularly after intravenous bolus injection of contrast agents, the looped and enlarged carotid arteries within the cavernous sinus can be nicely demonstrated by CT (Fig. 35).

Schloffer (1934) has demonstrated the typical finding of a dolichoectatic artery bulging into the cavernous sinus in a patient with the clinical signs of oculomotor nerve compression, pressure atrophy of the optic nerve and pressure atrophy of the first branch of the trigeminal nerve in a patient with optic atrophy in one eye and disk swelling in the other.

The frequent association of pain and dysaesthesia or hypaesthesia in patients with vascular third nerve palsies in the presence of gross dolichoectasia of the intracavernous portion of the internal carotid artery as well as its association with optic nerve compression by the supracavernous portion of the internal carotid artery in some cases adds further evidence for such a local compressive mechanism (Schildwächter and Unsöld 1987).

Fig. 16. Optic disk of a 43-year-old female with a 3-year history of progressive visual loss and an almost blind left eye due to an optic nerve sheath meningioma growing into the intracranial end of the optic canal (for CT findings see Fig. 37). There is chronic papilledema with severe optic atrophy and optociliary shunt vessels

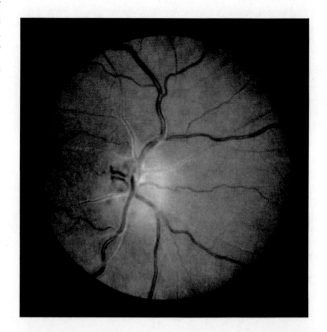

Fig. 17 a, b. Outer aspect (*a*) and right optic disk (*b*) of a 36-year-old female with a congenital optic nerve sheath meningioma and a blind right eye (for CT findings see Fig. 36). There are 4 mm of axial proptosis of the right eye (*a*) and total optic atrophy of the right optic disk (*b*)

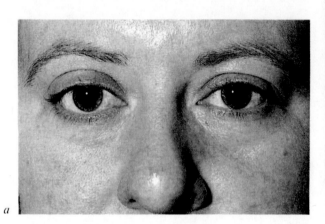

a

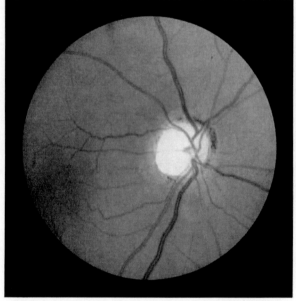

b

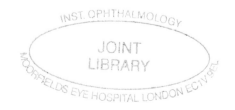

INST. OPHTHALMOLOGY
JOINT
LIBRARY
MOORFIELDS EYE HOSPITAL LONDON EC1V 9EL

21

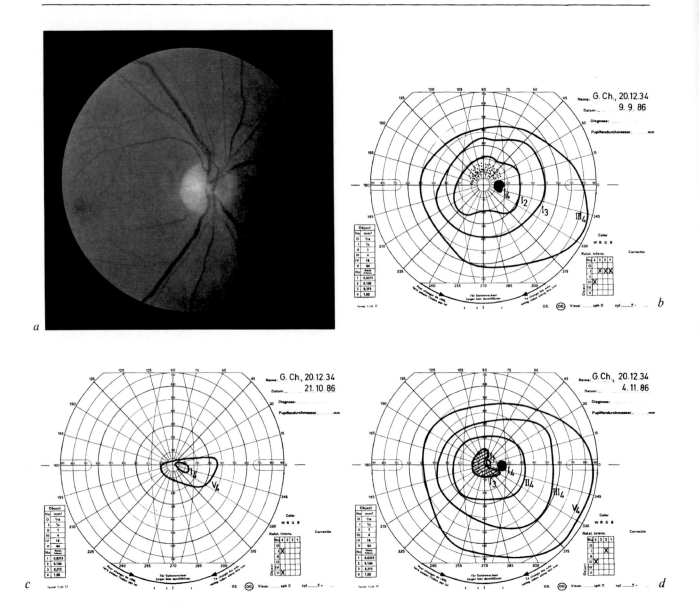

Fig. 18a–d. Optic disk (*a*) and sequential visual fields (*b–d*) of the right eye of a 52-year-old female with surgically confirmed optic nerve compression by a dolichoectatic right internal carotid artery. There is diffuse partial optic atrophy slightly more pronounced in the lower arcuate nerve fiber bundle (*a*). The picture was taken at the time when the central scotoma and incipient superior altitudinal field defect were detected (*b*). Severe concentric restriction occurred with increasing compression (*c*). After decompressive surgery there is considerable improvement (*d*). (For details see p. 87)

Fig. 19a–c. Right optic disk and computed visual fields of a 43-year-old male with surgically confirmed optic nerve compression by dolichoectasia of the right internal carotid artery. (For details see p. 99.) There is (*a*) diffuse optic atrophy of the right optic disk and (*b*) a marked, mainly temporal visual field defect (octopus program 31). Note the improvement of the visual field defect after decompressive surgery (*c*)

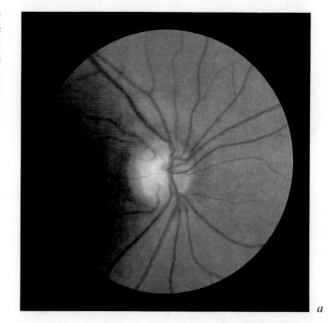

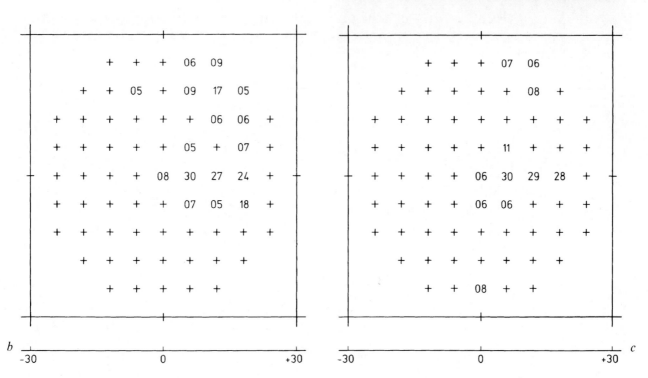

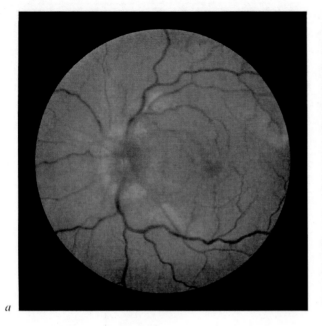

Fig. 20 a, b. Left optic disk of a 66-year-old female with surgically confirmed optic nerve compression by an ectatic left internal carotid artery within the optic canal (for details see p. 106). There is marked chronic papill-edema with optic atrophy (*a*). Papilledema resolved within 10 days after surgery (*b*) leaving marked diffuse optic atrophy

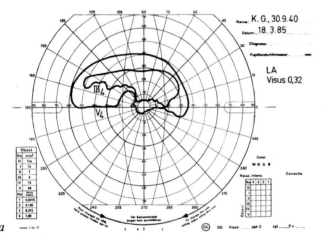

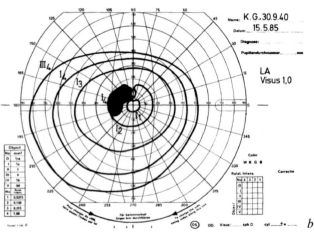

Fig. 21a, b. Preoperative (*a*) and postoperative (*b*) left visual field of a 45-year-old male with focal pneumosinus dilatans causing bone erosion of the medial and lower portions of the left optic canal. During surgery the optic nerve was observed to be pressed against the rigid dural fold crossing over the intracranial optic canal. Besides a central scotoma there is an almost complete inferior altitudinal visual field defect and constriction of the remaining superior visual field (*a*). After surgery (*b*) the visual field has recovered and there is only a paracentral scotoma probably due to occlusion of a retinal vessel. (For details see p. 117)

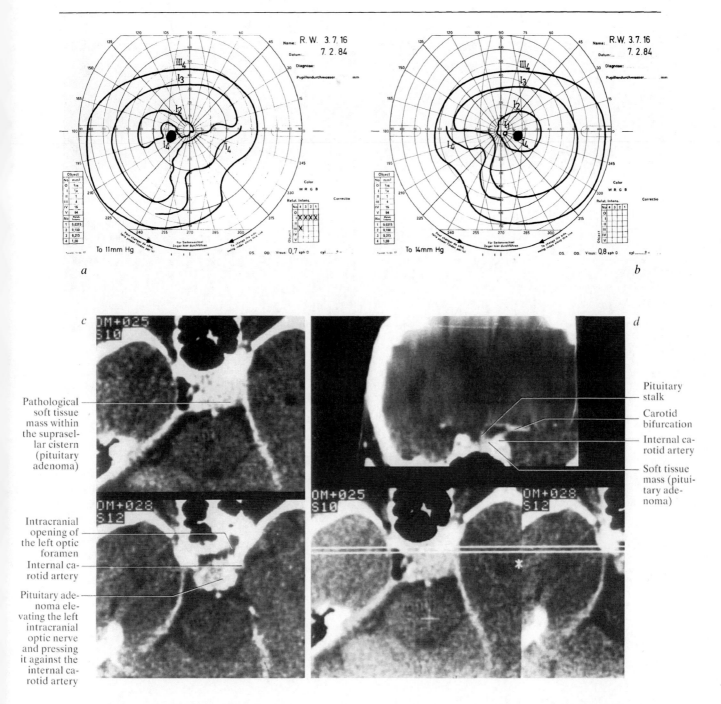

Pathological
soft tissue
mass within
the suprasel-
lar cistern
(pituitary
adenoma)

Intracranial
opening of
the left optic
foramen
Internal ca-
rotid artery

Pituitary ade-
noma ele-
vating the left
intracranial
optic nerve
and pressing
it against the
internal ca-
rotid artery

Pituitary
stalk

Carotid
bifurcation

Internal ca-
rotid artery

Soft tissue
mass (pitui-
tary ade-
noma)

Fig. 22a–d. Visual fields and CT findings in a 68-year-old male with a pituitary adenoma and moderate optic atrophy. Besides a moderate central scotoma there is mainly an inferior nasal visual field defect, which is more pronounced on the left (*a*) than on the right (*b*), corresponding to the suprasellar extension of the pituitary adenoma which elevates the optic nerves and presses them superiorly and laterally against the internal carotid artery and anterior clinoid process more marked on the left than on the right side (*c, d*). Axial sections (*c*) show extension of the abnormal hyperdense soft tissue mass into the suprasellar cistern which is more pronounced on the left side. Coronal computer reformation at the level of the intracranial optic canal (*d*) demonstrating the abnormal soft tissue creeping into the intracranial optic canal

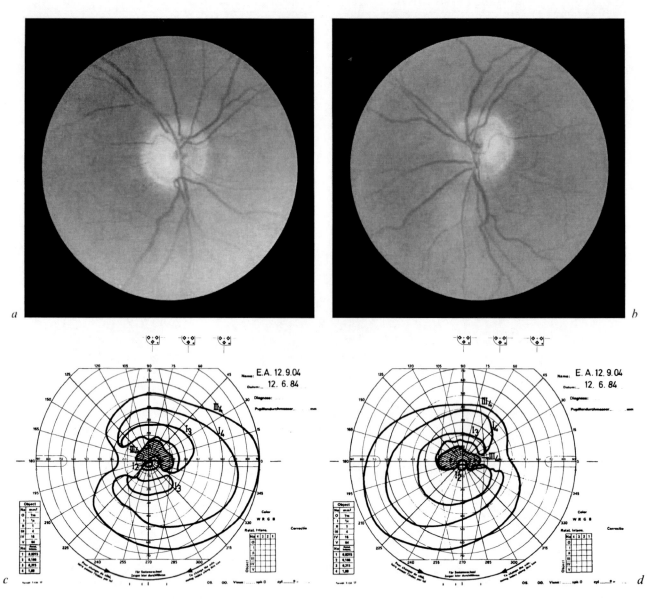

Fig. 23 a–d

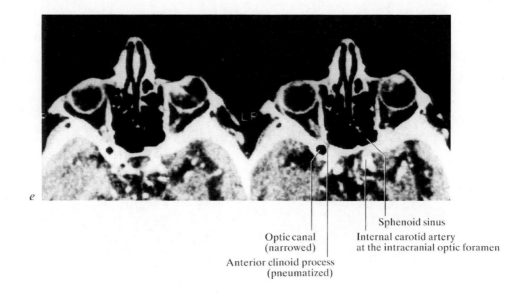

e

Sphenoid sinus

Optic canal
(narrowed)

Internal carotid artery
at the intracranial optic foramen

Anterior clinoid process
(pneumatized)

Fig. 23a–e. Optic disks of an 80-year-old female with slowly progressive optic
atrophy and cupping of the optic disk (*a, b*) and mainly superior paracentral
visual field defects (*c, d*), considered "characteristic" of glaucoma. The patient
had always normal intraocular pressure (about 15 mmHg), but considerable
bilateral dolichoectasia of the internal carotid artery in the presence of narrow
optic canals due to luxury pneumatization of the sphenoid sinus and lesser
wing of the sphenoid bone (*e*)

3.2
Visual Evoked Potentials in Optic Nerve Compression

M. Bach

The visual evoked potential (VEP) depends on an intact *function* of the entire optic pathway, i.e., from the optics of the eye up to the primary visual cortex. Diagnostic criteria are based on latency and amplitude of the VEP, sometimes its shape is also taken into account.

Pathophysiological Model

A simple model explains many of the pathological effects apparent in the VEP: Inflammatory lesions, causing demyelination of the optic nerve fibers, primarily lead to prolongation of the conduction time appearing as latency increase (Halliday 1976). Compression, causing partial blockade of conduction, primarily leads to amplitude reduction but may also be accompanied by increase in latency (Halliday et al. 1976; Röver et al. 1983), corresponding to the histological finding of demyelination in focal compressive optic nerve lesions.

Stimulation

Visual stimulation is performed by contrast reversal (about once per second) of a checkerboard pattern, presented on a TV-type display unit or by a projection system. High contrast (>90%) and high luminance (>10 cd/m²) should be used for clinical routine (Diener and Zimmermann 1985). We use a check size of 0.4°, higher values can be useful with poor visual acuity. Stimulation by unpatterned light flashes conveys little diagnostic information, as in normals it evokes a VEP with large variability in latency, amplitude and shape (Shearer et al. 1983). Correct refraction and correction is an indispensable precondition for reliable results (Sokol and Moskowitz 1981; Röver and Bach 1987).

Recording

A typical montage of the recording electrodes is 3 cm above the inion versus a midfrontal reference. Topographic representation based on multichannel recording has not found widespread acceptance so far; one of its drawbacks is the poor topographic resolution.

Normative Values

As the VEP is affected by a very large number of stimulation and recording parameters, standard values and normal ranges must be established in each laboratory (Shearer and Dustman 1980). The latency displays a remarkably high intra- and interindividual stability as compared to the high variability of the amplitude (John 1973; Yolton et al. 1983). The coefficient of variation is 5% for latency and about 50% for amplitude values.

Interocular Comparison

In compressive lesions distal to the chiasm, diagnostic reliability can be increased by comparison of the VEP-amplitude to stimulation of either eye, since in normal individuals the difference in amplitude does not exceed 20%.

Pattern-ERG

A pattern-evoked potential which can be measured at the corneal surface (Riggs et al. 1964; Lawwil 1984) has recently gained clinical interest: the pattern-ERG. Compared to the flash-evoked ERG it is of much lower amplitude (5 µV) and probably results from the activity of the retinal ganglion cells. It decreases with ganglion cell atrophy while the luminance-ERG remains. In acute blockage, the VEP is lost but the pattern-ERG remains until atrophy occurs (up to 3 months; Maffei and Fiorentini 1981). In acute optic neuritis, the VEP may be extinguished but the pattern-ERG is often not affected (Persson and Wanger 1984). The pattern-ERG is less dominated by central retina than the VEP. Even more than the VEP, the pattern-ERG depends on the sharpness of the retinal image.

Clinical Relevance

The VEP reflects the functional state of the visual pathway and therefore adds complementary information to that gained by modern imaging procedures such as CT and MR.

Due to the smaller relative normal range of latency compared to amplitude values, evoked potentials are a more reliable tool for detection of demyelinating lesions than for optic nerve compressions. However, clearcut amplitude reduction with little increase in latency most probably represents partial blockage of conduction and is caused either by acute compression or atrophy of the optic nerve fibers.

Amplitude reduction combined with latency increase does not yield more information than an objective correlate of some kind of optic nerve disease. Amplitude evaluation can be improved by interocular comparison.

Follow-up VEPs may substantiate a diagnosis of optic neuritis, since in most cases complete amplitude recovery occurs, but latency remains at pathologically high values for years.

Combined simultaneous recording of VEP and pattern-ERG allows better prognostic estimation of visual function after decompressive surgery: With pathologic VEP but intact pattern-ERG, a better result can be expected than if both VEP and pattern-ERG are pathologic (Kaufman et al. 1986).

Fig. 24. (*a*) Pre- and postoperative VEP in a patient with left optic nerve compression due to a focal pneumosinus dilatans (Case 6). Above: preoperative VEP. Right eye (RE): normal latency, amplitude low but within normal range. Left eye (LE): considerable reduction of amplitude to about 1/5 of normal value, latency above normal limits. Below: postoperative VEP. Right eye (RE): normal latency, amplitude increase compared to preoperative value up to a normal level. Left eye (LE): amplitude increase compared to preoperative value, reduction of latency compared to preoperative value, but still above normal limits.

Conclusion: The VEP-loss is in concordance with a compression of the visual pathway. This was confirmed during surgery. There was considerable improvement of visual function, reflected in the VEP-amplitude increase to stimulation of the left eye. We have no explanation for the increase of amplitude in the right eye

(*b*) Simultaneously recorded pattern-ERG and VEP of the left eye.

Finding: The pattern-ERG is normal (positive peak at 52 ms with an amplitude of 3.8 μV); the VEP shows considerable reduction of amplitude to about 1/5 of normal value, latency is above normal limits. Note widely differing latency of the VEP compared to Fig. 24a (top right), indicating poor reproducibility due to the considerable reduction of amplitude.

Conclusion: The normal pattern-ERG indicates that no massive ganglion cell lesion has occurred

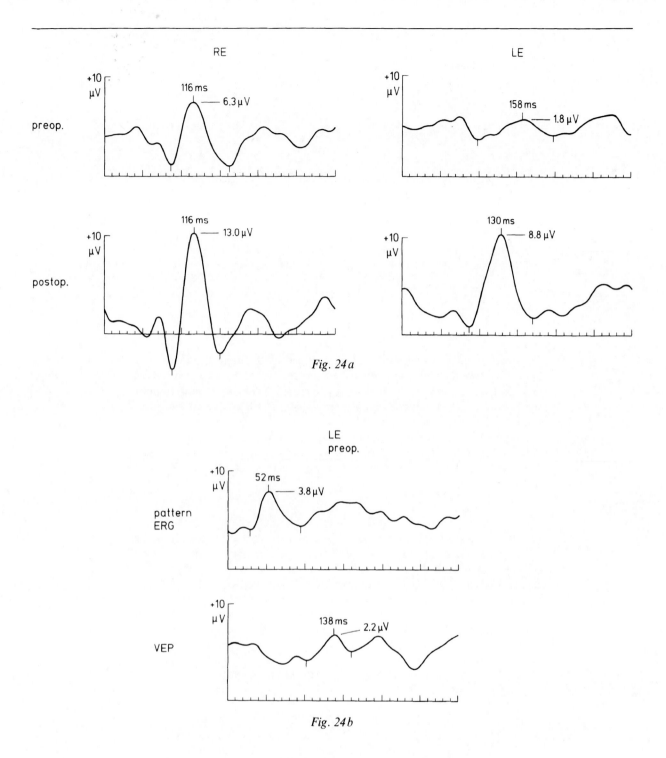

RE

LE

preop.

116 ms — 6.3 µV

158 ms — 1.8 µV

postop.

116 ms — 13.0 µV

130 ms — 8.8 µV

Fig. 24a

LE
preop.

pattern
ERG

52 ms — 3.8 µV

VEP

138 ms — 2.2 µV

Fig. 24b

RE

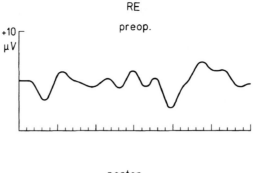

preop.

+10
µV

postop.

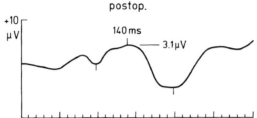

+10
µV

140 ms

3.1µV

Fig. 25. Pre- and postoperative VEP in a patient with surgically proven right optic nerve compression by a dolichoectatic carotid artery (Case 3). Above: preoperatively, no reproducible VEP can be recorded. Below: after decompressive surgery, VEP-amplitude has recovered but is still below normal limits, latency is also above normal limits.

Conclusion: The preoperative finding of strong amplitude reduction indicated most likely a compression of the optic nerve. This was confirmed during surgery. There was considerable improvement of visual function, reflected in the increase of VEP-amplitude

Fig. 26. (*a*) Pre- and postoperative VEP in a patient with surgically proven ▷ right optic nerve compression by a dolichoectatic internal carotid artery with considerable functional improvement after surgery without electrophysiological correlate (Case 1). Above: preoperative VEP. Right eye (RE): normal latency, amplitude low but within normal limits. Left eye (LE): normal latency and amplitude. Below: postoperative VEP. Right eye (RE): increased latency, amplitude low but within normal limits, no significant change compared to preoperative values. Left eye (LE): normal latency and amplitude, no change compared to preoperative values.

Conclusion: No electrophysiological correlate of the clinical improvement in visual function of the right eye

(*b*) Preoperative pattern-ERG and VEP of the same patient as in Fig. 26a. Above: preoperative pattern-ERG; below: simultaneously recorded VEP.

Finding: The pattern-ERG-amplitude (positive peak at 52 ms) of the right eye is lower than for the left eye but within normal limits.

Conclusion: No gross ganglion cell deterioration, indicating good prognosis for surgery

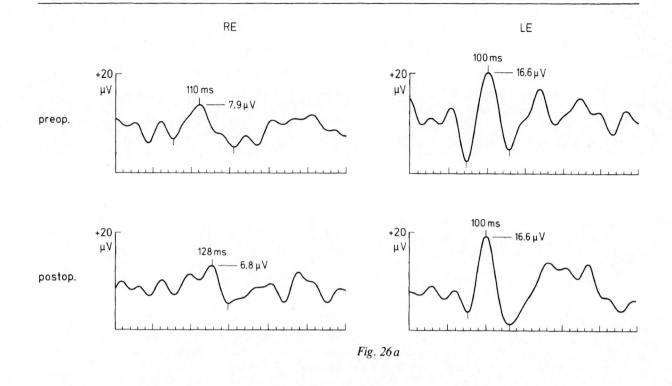

Fig. 26 a

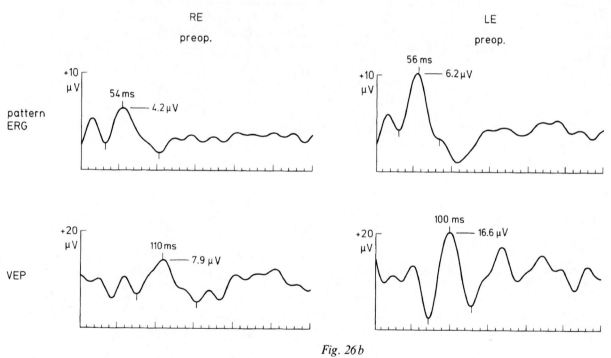

Fig. 26 b

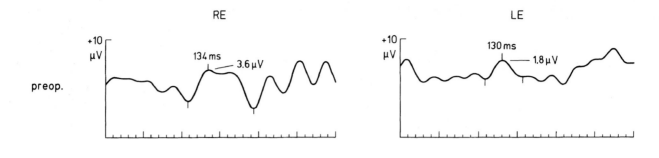

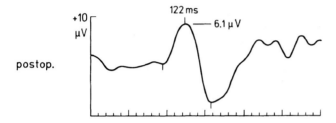

Fig. 27. Pre- and postoperative VEP in a patient with a surgically proven right optic nerve compression due to dolichoectatic internal carotid artery and a left pneumosinus dilatans causing narrowing of the left optic canal (Case 2). Above: preoperative VEP. For both eyes, latency is above normal limits, amplitude is below normal limits. Below: postoperative VEP. Right eye (RE): latency slightly above normal limits, amplitude low but within normal limits.

Conclusion: Preoperatively, the marked reduction of amplitude combined with a moderate latency increase points to blockage of conduction by compression rather than to an inflammatory disease. Surgery has led to functional improvement with a clear electrophysiological correlate

4

The Concept of Optic Nerve Compression by Dolichoectatic Arteries Revisited

The Literature and Why It Became Forgotten

R. Unsöld

The concept of dolichoectatic vessels of the anterior circle of Willis acting like space-occupying lesions that cause optic nerve compression at the optic canal dates back to the 19th century (Türk 1852; Knapp 1875; Michel 1877; Bernheimer 1981, and others). For a time, this concept was forgotten and was rediscovered on the basis of thorough post mortem examinations by Otto 1901; Liebrecht 1902; Behr 1910; Henschen 1911; Willbrand and Sänger 1931; Klieneberger 1913; Sattler 1920; Fuchs 1922; Mazzatesta 1925; Abelsdorf 1928; Alpers and Wolman 1931; Saphir 1933; Walsh 1957; Sacks and Lindenberg 1969; Lindenberg et al. 1973, and others.

The mechanism of compression observed during brain surgery was described by Caramazza 1932; Schloffer 1934; Sandford et al. 1935; Adson 1941; Yaskin and Schlezinger 1942; Tassman 1944; McLean and Ray 1947; Ley 1950; Parin 1951; Schmidt 1953; Ricci and Werner 1957; Bergaust 1963; Mitts and McQueen 1965; Matsuo et al. 1980, and others. Not even the fact that decompressive surgery had been documented to improve visual function in some patients (Sandford et al. 1935; Adson 1941; Ley 1950; Schmidt 1953; Ricci and Werner 1957; Matsuo et al. 1980) was able to save the concept of direct optic nerve compression by dolichoectatic vessels from being abandoned. Walsh and Hoyt (1969) after reviewing most of the literature conclude that "the direct effects of the sclerotic fusiform aneurysms or ectasias on the optic nerve in the region of the optic canal are probably less significant, but serve to compound the visual loss in some cases". Furthermore, the frequently acute onset of visual loss and the presence of atrophy in one eye and papilledema in the other eye, as described in several cases of "Foster-Kennedy Syndrome" in patients found at surgery and autopsy to have gross carotid artery disease, was interpreted as representing ischemic optic neuropathy, which was thought to be caused by occlusion of the ciliary arteries immediately behind the eyeball. The findings of dolichoectatic internal carotid arteries at surgery or autopsy in these patients was considered "incidental but important for the underlying vascular nature of visual dysfunction". The mechanism of vascular occlusion at the circle of Zinn was suspected to be embolization by atheromatous debris from the internal carotid arteries. In the 4th edition of Walsh and Hoyt's *Clinical Neuroophthalmology,* there is only very brief mention of dolichoectatic vessels being a possible cause of retrobulbar compressive optic neuropathies without optic disk swelling (Miller 1982).

The theory of direct optic nerve compression by dolichoectatic vessels was abandoned, despite surgical and autoptic evidence, probably for the following reasons:

1. Before computerized tomography was introduced, the condition could not be demonstrated in the living patient. Neither is there a correlation between calcifications of the carotid artery, as seen in conventional radiography, nor of the lumen of the arteries demonstrated by angiography (Knapp 1940; Saphir 1933; Walsh and Hoyt 1969). The vascular changes responsible for nerve compression in the absence of gross calcifications or stenosis lie within the vessel wall, which could not be visualized prior to thin section CT.

2. The results of decompressive neurosurgical intervention before the introduction of microsurgical techniques and special approaches in neurosurgery as well as further advances in anesthesiology were rather poor and associated with high morbidity and mortality rates. Furthermore, at that time craniotomy was usually done at a very late stage of the disease when severe optic atrophy had already developed and no significant functional improvement could possibly be expected.

3. A new disease entity referred to as "ischemic optic neuropathy" was discovered, which was thought to be due to ciliary artery occlusion. The latter could be demonstrated experimentally in monkeys at autopsy, which led to the assumption that this mechanism may have been the true and only cause of optic nerve disease, even in those patients with surgically or autoptically proven dolichoectatic vascular changes.

With thin section CT using appropriate examination techniques, the anatomic relationship of the internal carotid artery as a whole (wall and lumen) and the optic canal can be visualized, as well as the predisposing factors for optic nerve compression. Recognition of these details and simultaneous exclusion of other compressive lesions in the presence of clear clinical signs and symptoms of optic nerve compression (see Chap. 3) appear to be sufficient indication for microsurgical decompression. The typical clinical, radiological, and intraoperative findings in optic nerve compression by ectatic vessels as well as the functional results of decompressive surgery are demonstrated in cases 1–4 of the selected case reports.

These findings indicate not only the existence of this disease entity but also that decompression by microsurgical techniques may not only preserve but also improve visual function.

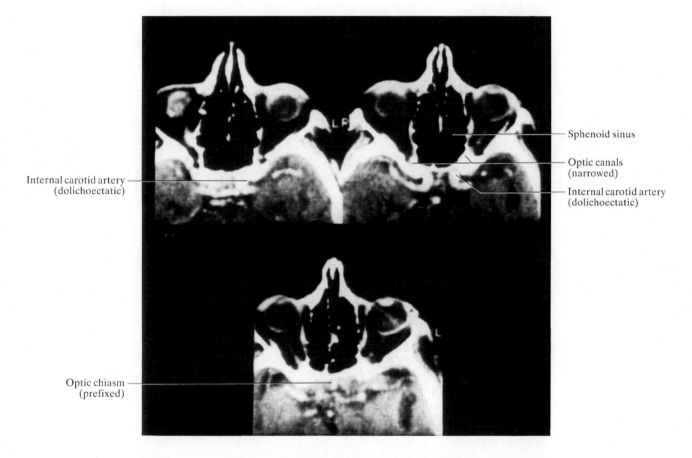

Fig. 28. Ectasia of both internal carotid arteries in a 76-year-old woman with progressive visual loss and optic atrophy. The ectatic internal carotid arteries reach into the intracranial end of the optic canals, the latter being narrowed by luxury pneumatization of the sphenoid sinus. The chiasm is in a prefixed position

5
Pneumosinus Dilatans –
Rarely Diagnosed and Poorly Understood

R. Unsöld

The term "pneumosinus dilatans" was coined by Benjamins in 1918 in his description of ballooning hyperpneumatization of the frontal sinus. The phenomenon of pathological pneumatization within the paranasal sinuses had been observed earlier (Mejyes 1898; Röpke 1905; Wittmak 1918). "Pneumosinus dilatans" was used later on for excessive pneumatization of individual or several paranasal sinuses or parts of individuals paranasal sinuses, with or without local compressive signs. It could be observed as an isolated finding or associated with various lesions, in particular meningiomas, hemangiomas, phacomatoses, and cerebral atrophy. After the early publications of Mejyes (1898), Benjamins (1918), Wittmak (1918), Feldmann (1923), Hayek (1926), and Leichner (1928), there was almost a boom of publications between 1930 and 1940 (Koch 1930; Schüller 1930; Bendesco 1932; Stanka 1933; Pages 1935; Killian 1939; Zange and Moser 1940; Agati 1940, and others). Later on, after a period of silence, the phenomenon of hyperpneumatization again became a subject of great interest, and between 1950 and 1956 a series of thorough discussions on the mechanism of pathological pneumatization and predisposing factors appeared, mainly in the ENT literature (Nötzel 1950; Kahler 1950; Oltersdorf 1953, 1954; Link and Handl 1954; Montresor 1954; Schlosshauer 1955; Püschel and Schlosshauer 1956). This resulted in the well-established diseases entity being represented in neuroradiological text books (Psenner 1963; Beutel and Tänzer 1963; Lombardi 1967; Lloyd 1975, and others). Then it was forgotten again, only to be partially rediscovered in the late 1970s and early 1980s (Leonardi 1976; Vine et al. 1976; Morrison et al. 1976; Kaufmann et al. 1977; Prott 1977; Hirst et al. 1979; Meyers and Burtschi 1980; Spoor et al. 1981; Hirst et al. 1982; Zoon et al. 1983; Morton et al. 1983; Morton 1983; Unsöld 1983; Hassler and Eggert 1985; Reicher et al. 1986).

In spite of these numerous publications, the phenomenon of pneumosinus dilatans of paranasal sinuses never became par-

39

ticularly popular. Excessive pneumatization of a frontal or maxillary sinus with outward bulging of the forehead or cheek in most cases can already be suspected on the basis of the patient's outer aspect. Pneumosinus dilatans of the ethmoid air cells or sphenoid sinus, however, may be difficult to diagnose. But these are the only forms that represent a serious threat to visual function due to possible compression of the anterior visual pathway. The observations of excessive pneumatization, mainly of the sphenoid sinus and lesser wing of the sphenoid bone in patients with visual loss, visual field defects, and optic atrophy, were published by a number of authors between 1932 and 1977 (Bendesco 1932; Stanka 1933; Agati and Bertolotti 1940; Jezegabel 1960; Lombardi 1967, 1968; Makialowitz 1969; Fels 1970; Williams et al. 1975; Sugita et al. 1977, and others). However, they seemed to have never actually reached the consciousness of most clinicians, who are primarily confronted with the presenting signs and symptoms. This was probably due to several factors:

1. Descriptions of pneumosinus dilatans were scattered over the ophthalmic, ENT, radiological, neurological and neurosurgical literature.

2. The diagnosis of sphenoid pneumosinus dilatans in particular was difficult to establish by conventional radiological methods and demonstration of the indirect signs of a compressive mechanism was almost impossible prior to the introduction of thin section CT.

3. The etiology and pathogenesis of pneumosinus dilatans were a matter of speculation and remained unsatisfactory to researchers and clinicians.

4. Neurosurgical publications on the mechanism revealed by exploratory surgery and presenting encouraging surgical results were scarce. Exploratory surgery was usually limited to the exclusion of suprasellar mass lesions or meningiomas en plaque. The mechanism of pneumosinus dilatans causing a tumor-like elevation of the planum sphenoidale or tuberculum sellae, or narrowing or erosion of the bony optic canal that resulted in compression of the optic nerve or chiasm remained unrecognized.

5. The considerable variations of pneumatization of the paranasal sinuses, particularly of the sphenoid sinus and lesser wing of the sphenoid bone, as known from many text-books (Leicher 1928; Koch 1930; Killian 1939; Oltersdorf 1954; Mayer 1959; Pfings 1964; Dune et al. 1975; Fuchioka and Young 1978, and others) caused uncertainty whether luxury pneumatization in an individual case was physiological or already pathological.

Thin section CT with computer reformations using appropriate examination techniques in many cases provides, if not definitive proof, at least a strong suspicion of optic nerve compression. This is because the hyperpneumatization can be easily visualized and another compressive lesion such as a parasellar or suprasellar neoplasm can be ruled out. Using thin section CT and special computer reformations, narrowing and erosion of the optic canal can easily be demonstrated. This had been difficult to do by conventional radiological techniques that require special skills, as pointed out by Beutel and Tänzer (1963). They described the diameter of the bony optic canal as almost always subnormal in patients with hyperpneumatization of the lesser wing of the sphenoid bone. They also pointed out that in patients with a pneumatized anterior clinoid process, the air cell within the clinoid on the classic radiological views of the optic canal after Rhese may appear as a well-defined lumen the size of a normal optic canal. Even the experienced neuroradiologist may mistake it for the optic canal, having missed the true optic canal which may show a slit-like reduction of its diameter or bone erosion (Fig. 78). The lack of familiarity on the part of the clinician, especially the ophthalmologist and neurologist, who are usually the first to be confronted with the symptomatology, as well as the neuroradiologist, may account for the view that pneumosinus dilatans is an extremely rare condition, as is stated in the radiologic text books. Selz (1979) and others who reviewed larger numbers of patients with pneumosinus dilatans of the sphenoid bone have emphasized that this entity is undoubtedly diagnosed less often than it actually exists.

What are the clinical signs and symptoms of pneumosinus dilatans of the ethmoid or sphenoid sinus which require that this entity be radiologically visualized or excluded? The most frequent complaint are headaches, which are usually projected in the center of the head, the orbital, or occipital region. These headaches can be severe, as was pointed out by Schlosshauer (1956), Selz (1970), Reicher et al. (1986), and others. Compression of the optic nerves usually in the area of the optic canal may cause visual loss (Agati and Bertolotti 1940; Jezegabel 1960; Lombardi 1967; Lombardi et al. 1968; Makialowitz 1969; Williams et al. 1975; Sugita 1977; Unsöld 1983; Hassler and Eggert 1985; Spoor et al. 1981; Reicher et al. 1986, and others), visual field defects (Agati and Bertolotti 1940; Jezegabel 1960; Williams et al. 1975; Lombardi 1967; Lombardi et al. 1968; Makialowitz 1969; Unsöld 1983; Reicher et al. 1986), papilledema and optic atrophy and cannot be differentiated by clinical means from other compressive lesions in this area such as aneurysms, ectatic vessels, and small meningiomas. Rarely, there is associated paresis of an oculomotor, abducent, trigeminal or vestibulocochlear nerve (Selz 1970). Pneumosinus dilatans of the ethmoid air cells or sphenoid bone has been described, for instance, by Agati and Bertolotti (1946), Agati (1946), Montresor (1954), Petereit (1975), Morton (1983), and others, but is less frequent than hyperpneumatizations of the frontal and maxillary sinus (Morrison et al. 1976; Vine et al. 1976; Meyers and Burtschi 1980, and others). Bone erosion, usually in the area of the roof of the sphenoid sinus and around the optic canal, has been observed (Sugita et al. 1977; Kaufmann et al. 1977; Reicher et al. 1986) and may cause, apart from optic nerve compression, cerebral spinal fluid fistulas that occur spontaneously or after surgery of lesions in the ethmoid or sphenoid sinuses (Fig. 45). The character of visual loss may vary. Its onset can be acute, intermittent, or slowly progressive, it may be stationary for quite some time at some stage and then may suddenly progress, as was pointed out by Lombardi et al. (1968) and others. We observed a young man who experienced only a few episodes of blurred vision, after which he had no symptoms. Computerized tomography showed a marked unilateral pneumatization of the lesser wing of the sphenoid bone, the aerocele reaching far up into the suprasellar cistern. This pneumosinus caused intermittent optic nerve compression for a short time only and – probably by further expansion – was spontaneously "decompressing" the optic nerve (Fig. 44). In rare cases, compression of the pituitary gland by the pneumatocele may cause endocrine disturbances such as galactorrhea or mild hypopituitarism (Lombardi et al. 1968; Reicher et al. 1986).

The pathogenesis of excessive pneumatization in pneumosinus dilatans remains unknown. Certain features and associations with other pathological conditions seem to allow some speculation. The overwhelming preference of males between 20 and 40 years of age, as well as secondary pneumatization especially of the frontal sinuses, which is frequently observed in acromegalic patients, indicates that a hormonal factor is involved. Association with meningiomas has frequently been described and is known as "blistering" and as being associated with sclerotic bone changes of the planum sphenoidale or tuberculum sellae (Olivecrona 1927; Schüller 1930; Decker 1960; Psenner 1963; Beutel and Tänzer 1963; Lombardi et al. 1968; Wiggly et al. 1975; Leonardi and Fabris 1976; Hirst et al. 1979, 1982, and others). Other pathological conditions associated with focal pneumosinus dilatans are hemangiomas (Mayer 1959; Süsse 1964), particularly in connection with systemic diseases such as

Klippel-Trenaunay-Weber syndrome or Sturge-Weber syndrome, Recklinghausen's disease, and other phacomatoses (Psenner 1963; Weikmann 1958; Spoor et al. 1981). Furthermore, association of hyperpneumatization is observed with cerebral atrophy and long-lasting cerebral spinal fluid shunting procedures and in patients with a history of basal meningoencephalitis (Kaufmann 1970). Tissue pressure (Nötzel 1950), intracranial pressure (Güttner 1942), and circulatory factors (Süsse 1964) have been discussed as possible influences on the process of pneumatization.

A number of publications have dealt with local sinus disease being the basis of hyperpneumatization, particularly intermittent occlusion of the ostea by chronic swelling of the mucosa which causes a valve mechanism that leads to differences between the pressure within the affected sinus and the atmospheric pressure (Hayek 1926; Killian 1939; Zange and Moser 1940; Montresor 1954; Oltersdorf 1953, 1954; Fleischer 1956; Sugita et al. 1977; Mayer-Breiting 1978; Mayers and Burtschi 1980; Zoom et al. 1983; Reicher et al. 1986). These mechanisms have been extensively discussed by Kahler (1950), Oltersdorf (1953, 1954), Schlosshauer (1956), Ungerecht (1964), and others. The findings of pathological mucosa with chronic inflammatory signs and closure of the ostea in several patients have been taken as indications of a valve-like mechanism. During surgery both increased and decreased pressure were found within the enlarged paranasal sinus. Any difference between the atmospheric pressure and the pressure within the pneumosinus has been thought to represent a stimulus for pneumatization and bone resorption. It remains unclear whether the finding of partially or completely occluded ostea is primary or secondary to the hyperpneumatization (Ungerecht 1964). In our experience with about 24 patients with hyperpneumatization of the sphenoid sinus and lesser wing of the sphenoid bone, almost all of them had a history of allergic rhinitis.

In summary, there are most likely several factors that contribute to pathological pneumatization: hormonal factors, the influence of pressure differences between the pressure within the sinus and the atmospheric pressure, tissue pressure of the surrounding brain, its absence in cerebral atrophy, as well as possible pressure increases caused by local tumors. It cannot be ruled out that local irritation of the periosteum or circulatory particularities in the neighborhood of tumors may also influence pneumatization. Pressure measurements within the sinuses (Schlosshauer 1956 and others) and the observation of transient visual loss under conditions associated with atmospheric pressure decrease (Sugita 1977) do in fact confirm the hypothesis that a valve-like mechanism and pressure differences are important pathogenetic factors in pathological pneumatization. The therapy for pneumosinus dilatans causing signs of compression depends on both the underlying cause of hyperpneumatization and the kind of compressive signs and symptoms.

In the presence of a meningioma with secondary "blistering", surgical treatment of the meningioma is usually necessary.

In cases of nerve compression with visual loss or paresis, surgical decompression is usually indicated. In cases without clear signs of nerve compression of only intermittent symptomatology or very severe degrees of optic atrophy it may be sufficient to have a fenestration of the sinus to the nose performed by the ENT surgeon. The typical clinical and radiological signs of pneumosinus dilatans of the sphenoid bone resulting in optic nerve compression as well as the surgical results are demonstrated in Cases 5–6 (p. 111–123).

Figs. 29, 30. Hyperpneumatization of the sphenoid sinus and lesser wings of ▷ the sphenoid bones in a 63-year-old man with progressive bilateral visual loss without optic atrophy. The slightly ectatic internal carotid arteries are situated right at the intracranial opening of the optic canal (Fig. 29). There is luxury pneumatization causing elevation and bone erosion of the floor of both optic canals (coronal computer reformation, Fig. 30)

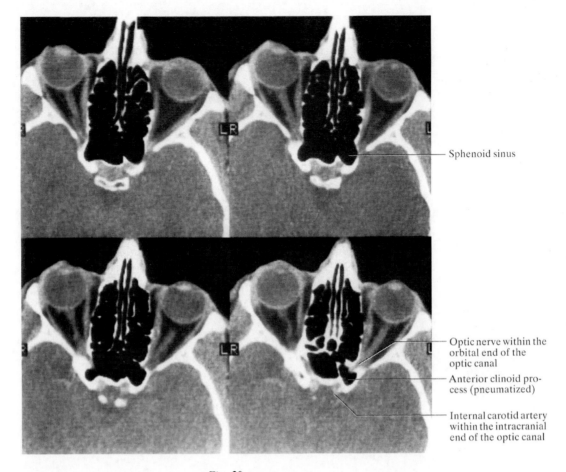

Sphenoid sinus

Optic nerve within the
orbital end of the
optic canal

Anterior clinoid pro-
cess (pneumatized)

Internal carotid artery
within the intracranial
end of the optic canal

Fig. 29

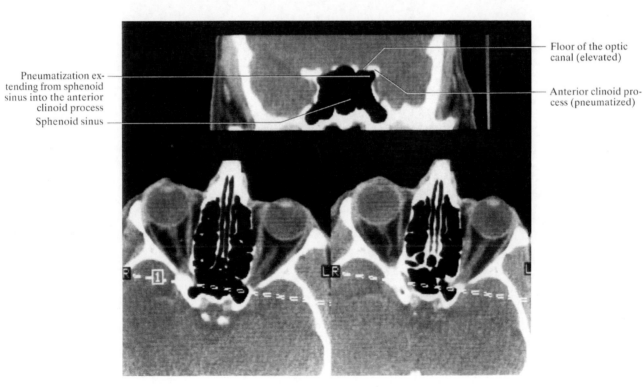

Floor of the optic
canal (elevated)

Anterior clinoid pro-
cess (pneumatized)

Pneumatization ex-
tending from sphenoid
sinus into the anterior
clinoid process

Sphenoid sinus

Fig. 30

6
CT Findings of Compressive Lesions at the Optic Canal

R. Unsöld, G. Greeven

Due to the topographical peculiarities around the optic canal, which are described in Chap. 2, even very small mass lesions or moderate changes of local structures may cause optic nerve compression and eventually blindness. In the past, such small lesions often could not be visualized by conventional radiographic methods, including polytomography and angiography. The introduction of thin section CT has considerably improved the evaluation of small mass lesions, hyperpneumatization of the sphenoid bone, and alterations of the local soft tissue structures, particularly the internal carotid arteries. CT has remained the method of choice for radiological evaluation of this region. It must be recognized, however, that to visualize or rule out small lesions in particular, specific techniques of examination as well as a thorough knowledge of the normal anatomy and its physiological variations are necessary to avoid false negative results or overinterpretations.

The optimal plane for the basic series of axial thin sections (1–2 mm) should be chosen at an angle of −10° to −15° to the orbital metal baseline (Fig. 3). In this plane the optic nerves are usually visualized within the optic canals as well as in the neighboring orbital and intracranial portion.

Paraxial computer reformations parallel and at 90° to the course of the optic canal and viewed with a bone window give further information on the canal's length, width, configuration, on bone erosion, hyperostosis, and on the degree of pneumatization; they are a satisfactory substitute for conventional topography in the projection after Rhese (Fig. 32). Soft tissue changes around the canal are to be assessed using a soft tissue window, and even very small tumors in the suprasellar cistern may be detected by cisternography with water soluble contrast media applied by lumbar puncture. This technique increases the sensitivity by increasing the density differences of the lesion and the surrounding tissues and media. Even small meningiomas attached to the dura may thus become visualized as filling defects within the suprasellar cistern, which appear white due to the dense contrast medium within the cerebral spinal fluid (Figs. 36 and 37).

Particularly for the evaluation of optic nerve compression caused by a dolichoectatic internal carotid artery or a pneumosinus, it is most important to check for possible predisposing factors such as the degree of pneumatization of the sphenoid sinus and anterior clinoid process, the configuration of the optic canal, the anatomic relationship of the internal carotid artery and optic canal, and the position of the optic chiasm. It therefore seems advisable to use a routine "check list" of details which need to be considered in the evaluation of compressive lesions. First, it is necessary to view all the axial sections in the vicinity of the optic foramen to evaluate the course and anatomic relationship, for instance, of the internal carotid artery and the optic canal. Additional information can usually be gained from special computer reformations through the optic canal.

Important details to be checked are:

1. Configuration, diameter, and quality of the bony walls of the optic canal viewed with a bone window (tortuous? narrowed? hyperostosis? bone erosion? pneumatization? floor of the canal elevated?).

2. Position, course, and caliber of the internal carotid artery and its relationship with the different portions of the optic canal as well as the appearance of the cavernous sinus. (How deep does the vessel reach into the canal? Relationship of the internal carotid artery to the intracranial end of the optic canal? Enlargement of the cavernous sinus? Configuration and caliber of the internal carotid artery?) Configuration and caliber of the internal carotid artery within the cavernous sinus may be defined by intravenous bolus injection of contrast medium if it is not already defined by calcifications within the vessel wall.

3. Position of the chiasm (prefixed? postfixed?).

4. Suprasellar cistern (well or ill defined? soft tissue density?) questionable findings may require cisternography (filling defect?).

Since the visual outcome in compressive lesions mainly depends on the early diagnosis of the lesion, visualization of minor abnormalities is of great importance. Radiological assessment has definitive limitations and almost always leaves some degree of uncertainty, since the radiological findings, particularly in small lesions, cannot reveal more than indirect signs of a compressive mechanism. The entire anatomy of the optic canal and surrounding structures must be analyzed. One single sign, such as the diameter of the optic canal or the internal carotid artery, if not grossly pathological, is usually not sufficient for a "diagnosis". At most, this would be no more than a strong suspicion. The indication for exploratory or decompressive surgery therefore needs to be based on both clinical and radiological findings. Sometimes, very similar radiological findings may be encountered in patients with and without clinical signs of optic nerve compression, and the degree of pressure tolerance varies considerably among individuals.

A very small intracanalicular meningioma may not be detectable at all, even by an optimal examination technique, unless it extends into the suprasellar cistern and causes a filling defect visualized by cisternography or causes characteristic changes of the adjacent bone ("blistering", hyperostosis). It might therefore make sense to go ahead with exploratory surgery in patients who show progressive clinical signs of optic nerve compression despite normal radiological findings.

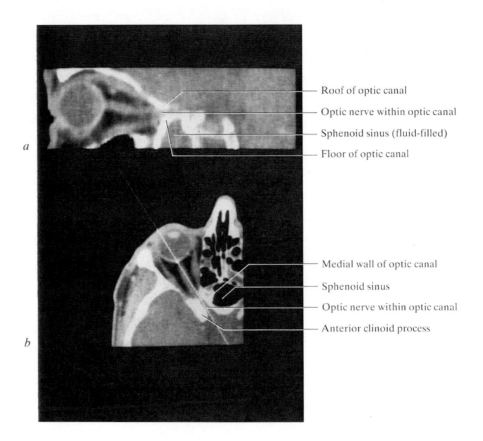

Roof of optic canal

Optic nerve within optic canal

Sphenoid sinus (fluid-filled)

Floor of optic canal

Medial wall of optic canal

Sphenoid sinus

Optic nerve within optic canal

Anterior clinoid process

a

b

Fig. 31 a–d

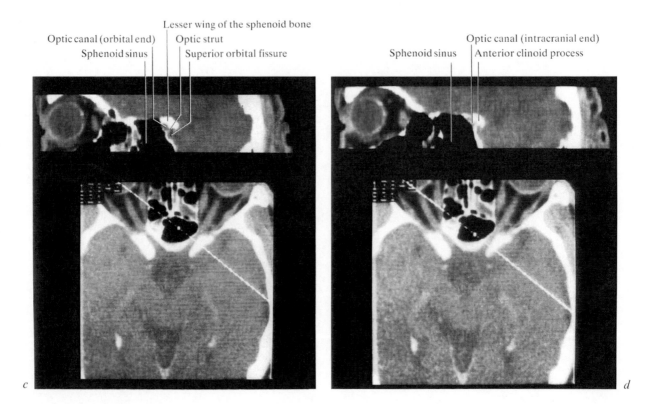

Lesser wing of the sphenoid bone

Optic canal (orbital end)   Optic strut

Sphenoid sinus   Superior orbital fissure

Optic canal (intracranial end)

Sphenoid sinus   Anterior clinoid process

c

d

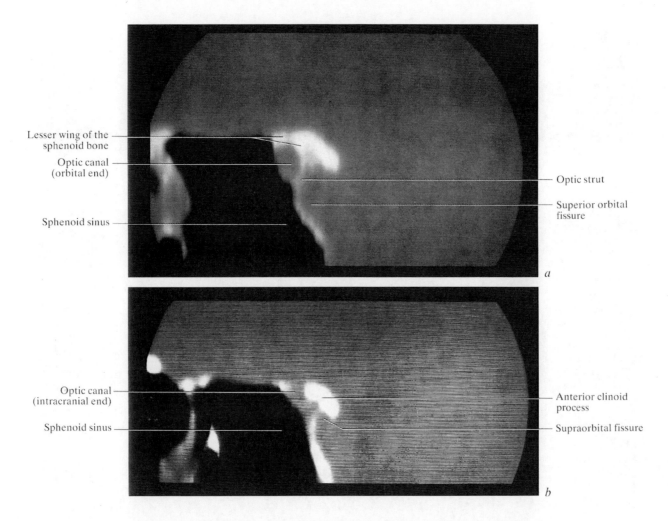

Lesser wing of the sphenoid bone

Optic canal (orbital end)

Sphenoid sinus

Optic strut

Superior orbital fissure

a

Optic canal (intracranial end)

Sphenoid sinus

Anterior clinoid process

Supraorbital fissure

b

Fig. 32a, b. Magnification of the computer reformations of Fig. 31c, d. The bony margins of the optic canal and superior orbital fissure are well visualized

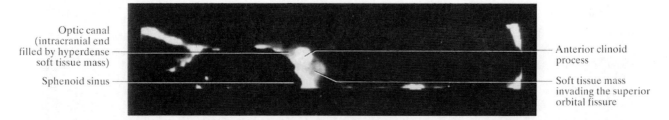

Optic canal (intracranial end filled by hyperdense soft tissue mass)

Sphenoid sinus

Anterior clinoid process

Soft tissue mass invading the superior orbital fissure

Fig. 33. Computer reformation perpendicular to the intracranial end of the optic canal in a patient with intracranial extension of an optic nerve sheath meningioma. There is hyperdense abnormal soft tissue around the hyperostotic anterior clinoid process. Note also hyperostosis of the neighboring wall of the sphenoid sinus

◁ Fig. 31a–d. Normal axial CT-sections. (a) 1.5 mm, near −10° to −15° to OMBL and standard computer reformations (above) parallel (b) and perpendicular to the orbital (c) and cranial (d) end of the optic canal. Plane of section is indicated on axial sections (below)

51

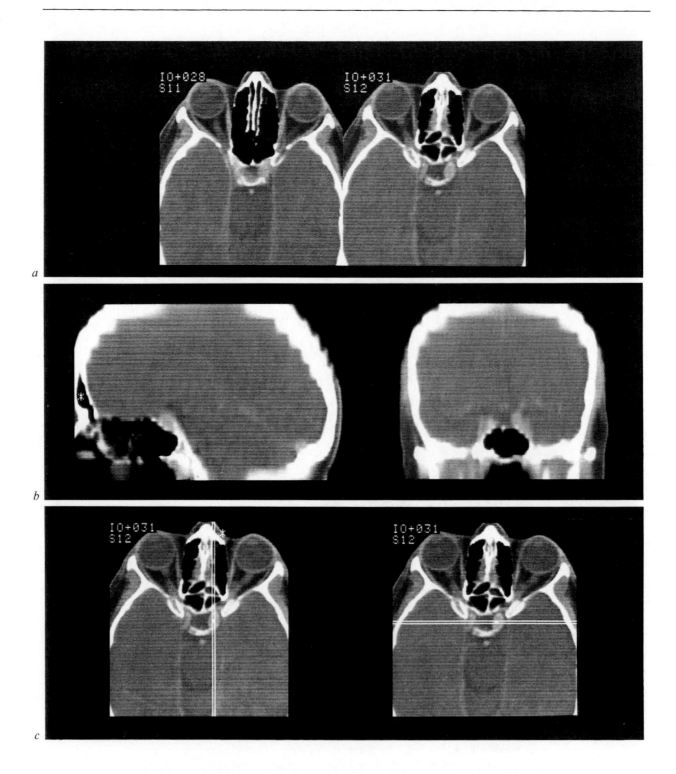

Fig. 34a–c. Aneurysm of the left internal carotid artery. (*a*) Sequential axial sections through the suprasellar cistern. A well-delineated oval zone of higher density occupies the left anterior corner of the suprasellar cistern. (*b*) Above: Parasagittal computer reformation. A well-defined roundish lesion of increased density is shown in the suprasellar cistern. Below: Plane of reformation. (*c*) Above: Coronal computer reformation. The well-delineated lesion is continuous with the left internal carotid and left middle cerebral arteries. Below: Plane of reformation (From Unsöld et al. 1982)

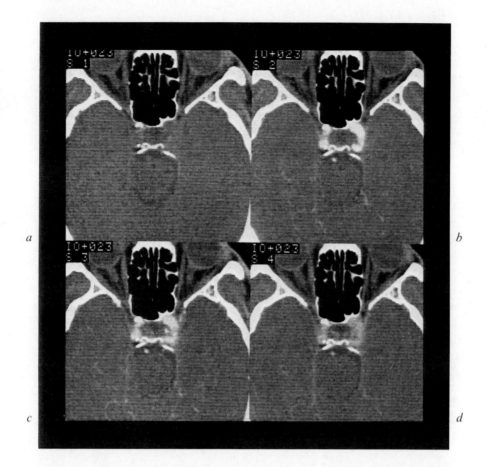

Fig. 35a–d. Intracavernous ectasia of the carotid artery causing a sudden onset of partial third nerve palsy with pupillary involvement. Sequential axial CT sections before and after bolus injection of contrast medium (upper left earliest scan, lower right latest). (*a*) Before contrast: there is only moderate enlargement of the left cavernous sinus, which does not allow differentiation between a possible soft tissue mass or an enlarged internal carotid artery (*b–d*). After bolus injection of contrast medium; the enhanced left internal carotid artery appears tortuous and markedly ectatic, causing distention of the left cavernous sinus, probably compressing the third cranial nerve within the cavernous sinus. On later scans (*c, d*) the contrast medium fades out. (From Unsöld et al. 1982.) Visualization of gross ectasia of the intracavernous portion of the internal carotid artery increases the probability of optic nerve compression by the supraclinoid portion of the same vessel in a patient with the clinical signs of nerve compression

Fig. 36a–d. Congenital optic nerve sheath meningioma in a 39-year-old woman ▷
with a blind right eye, total optic atrophy, and 4 mm of axial proptosis. There
was a slight temporal visual field defect in the left eye. The axial section through
the lower half of the right optic canal shows a thickened optic nerve, the
posterior portion of which is almost completely calcified (*a*), on the higher
axial section (*b*) focal hyperpneumatization around the right optic canal extending towards the planum sphenoidale is visualized. This represents "blistering"
in the vicinity of the intracranial portion of the meningioma growing en plaque
along the dura and partially obliterating the suprasellar cistern. Axial sections
through the lower (*c*) and higher (*d*) suprasellar cistern after application of
contrast medium by lumbar puncture (cisternography). There are considerable
filling defects (dark) around the right intracranial nerve and within the anterior
portion of the suprasellar cistern (light), extending up to the planum sphenoidale, as could be verified during surgery. Note focal pneumatization around
the optic canal. For clinical pictures see Fig. 19a, b

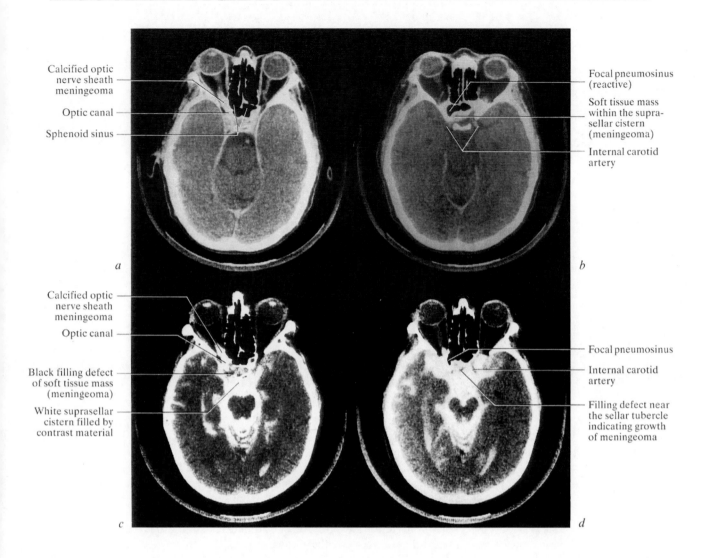

Calcified optic nerve sheath meningeoma

Optic canal

Sphenoid sinus

Focal pneumosinus (reactive)

Soft tissue mass within the suprasellar cistern (meningeoma)

Internal carotid artery

a

b

Calcified optic nerve sheath meningeoma

Optic canal

Black filling defect of soft tissue mass (meningeoma)

White suprasellar cistern filled by contrast material

Focal pneumosinus

Internal carotid artery

Filling defect near the sellar tubercle indicating growth of meningeoma

c

d

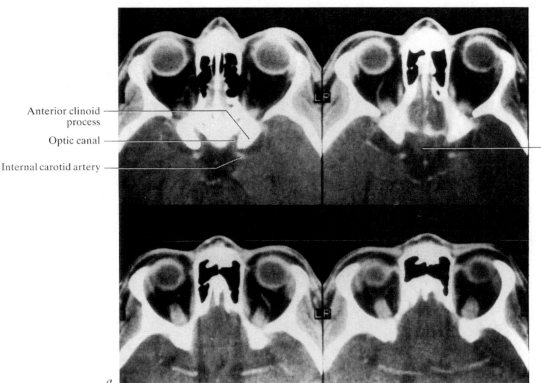

Anterior clinoid process

Optic canal

Internal carotid artery

Anterior suprasellar cistern (ill defined)

a

Fig. 37a–c. A 43-year-old woman with a 3-year history of progressive visual loss, chronic papilledema with progressive optic atrophy and optociliary shunt vessels. The left eye was almost blind, there was no functional loss in the right eye. Axial CT sections through the optic canal, suprasellar cistern and chiasm [(*a*) upper left lowest, lower right highest section]: the optic canal appears normal, the suprasellar cistern is ill defined, but it is uncertain whether this is due to the prefixed chiasm or the presence of pathological soft tissue. Cisternography of the same patient (*b*) at the intracranial end of the optic canal. There is a solid dark filling defect within the suprasellar cistern (lower left and lower right) representing pathological soft tissue. Coronal computer reformation (*c,* above) through the intracranial end of the optic canal showing the dark filling defect within the left optic canal extending superiorly. Plane of section is indicated on axial sections (below)

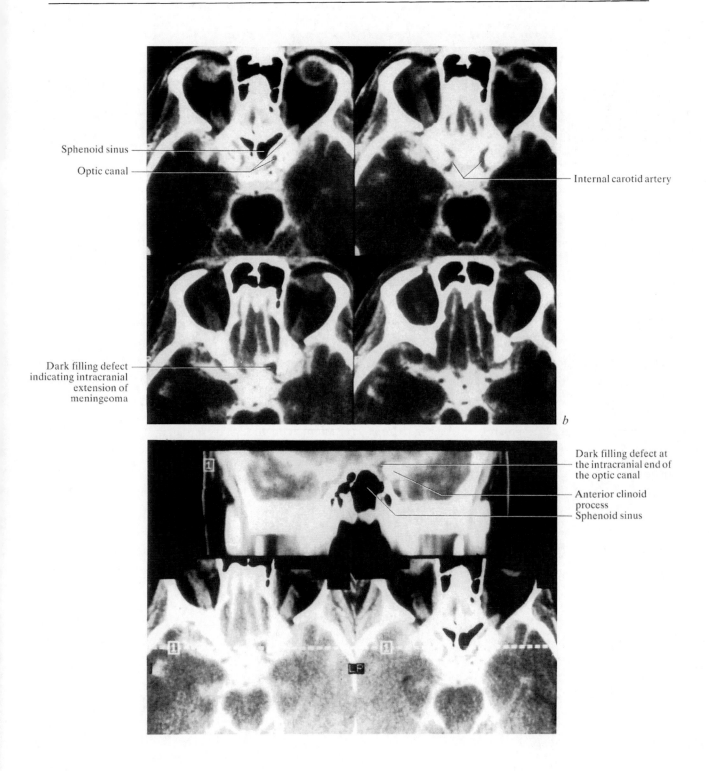

Sphenoid sinus

Optic canal

Internal carotid artery

Dark filling defect indicating intracranial extension of meningeoma

Dark filling defect at the intracranial end of the optic canal

Anterior clinoid process

Sphenoid sinus

b

Fig. 37b, c

57

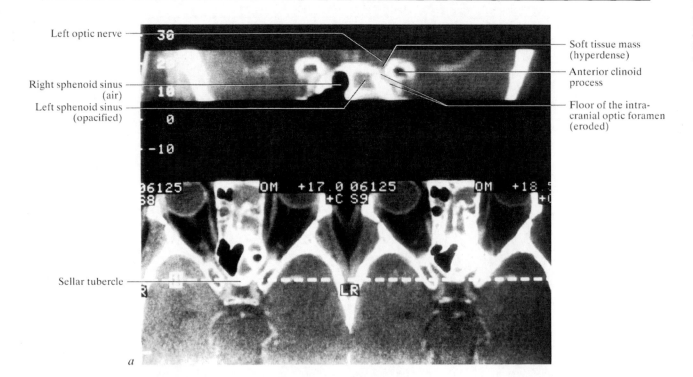

Left optic nerve

Right sphenoid sinus (air)

Left sphenoid sinus (opacified)

Soft tissue mass (hyperdense)

Anterior clinoid process

Floor of the intra-cranial optic foramen (eroded)

Sellar tubercle

a

Fig. 38a–c. Carcinoma of the ethmoid air cells extending into the left sphenoid sinus and eroding the left optic canal. It had infiltrated the left optic nerve causing progressive visual loss. Coronal CT reformation through the intracranial end of the optic canal (above, *a*). The left sphenoid sinus is filled with soft tissue, the floor of the left optic canal is eroded. Plane of section indicated on axial sections (below). Paraxial computer reformation perpendicular to the intracranial opening of the right (*b*) and left (*c*) optic canals (above) using a bone window. Plane of section indicated on axial sections (below). The right optic canal is well defined above the air-filled right sphenoid sinus. The left sphenoid sinus is filled with soft tissue and its lateral wall shows bone erosion. There is also pathological soft tissue around the left anterior clinoid process

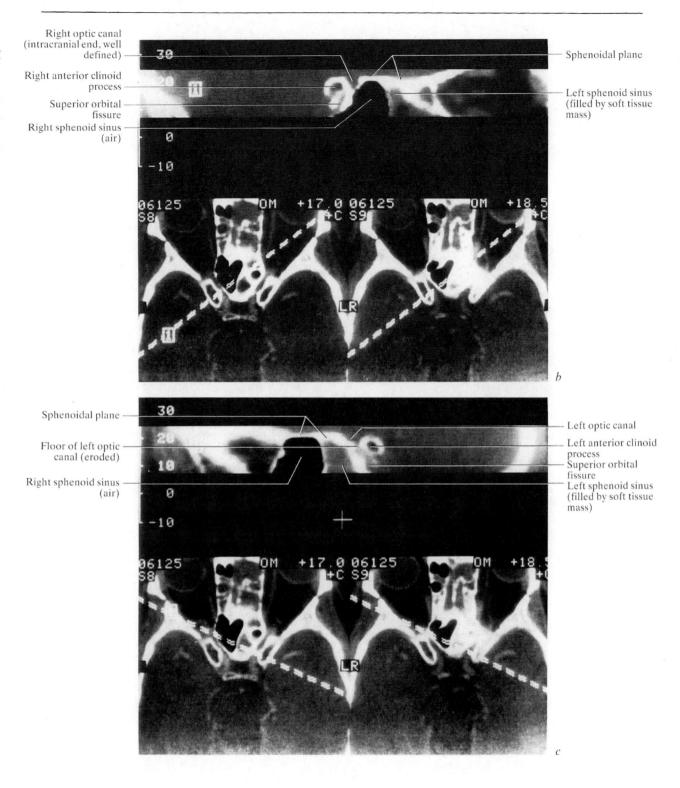

Right optic canal (intracranial end, well defined)

Right anterior clinoid process

Superior orbital fissure

Right sphenoid sinus (air)

Sphenoidal plane

Left sphenoid sinus (filled by soft tissue mass)

b

Sphenoidal plane

Floor of left optic canal (eroded)

Right sphenoid sinus (air)

Left optic canal

Left anterior clinoid process

Superior orbital fissure

Left sphenoid sinus (filled by soft tissue mass)

c

Fig. 38b, c

59

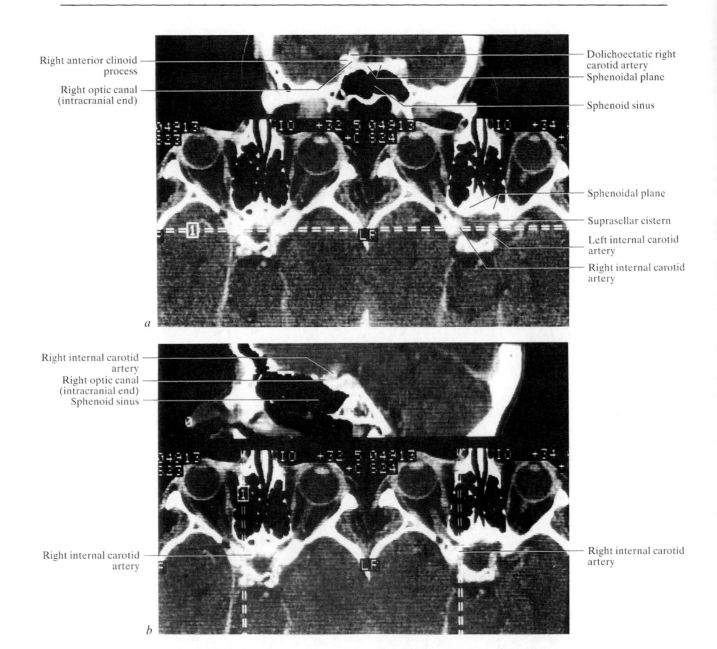

Right anterior clinoid process

Right optic canal (intracranial end)

Dolichoectatic right carotid artery

Sphenoidal plane

Sphenoid sinus

Sphenoidal plane

Suprasellar cistern

Left internal carotid artery

Right internal carotid artery

a

Right internal carotid artery

Right optic canal (intracranial end)

Sphenoid sinus

Right internal carotid artery

Right internal carotid artery

b

Fig. 39a, b. Dolichoectasia of the right internal carotid artery in a 67-year-old woman with severe visual loss and optic atrophy. Coronal computer reformation (*a*, above) through the intracranial optic canals demonstrating the dolichoectatic vessel. The right internal carotid artery reaches into the optic canal (axial section below, lower left). The intracranial end of the optic canal is almost filled by the ectatic vessel. Paraxial computer reformation (*b*, above) parallel to the right carotid siphon demonstrating the dolichoectatic internal carotid artery

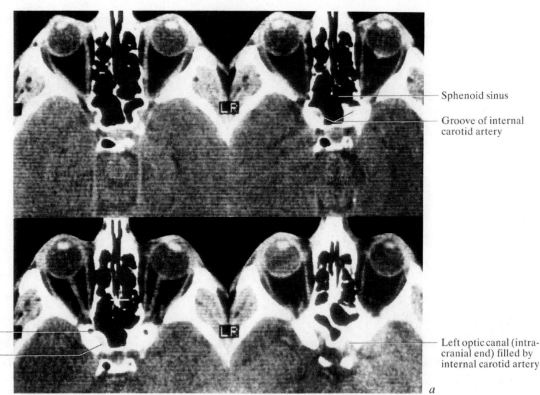

Sphenoid sinus

Groove of internal
carotid artery

Anterior clinoid
process (pneumatized)

Groove of internal
carotid artery elevating
floor of the optic canal

Left optic canal (intra-
cranial end) filled by
internal carotid artery

a

Fig. 40a–e. Moderate ectasia of the left internal carotid artery in the presence
of luxury pneumatization of the sphenoid sinus causing narrowing and a tortuous course of both optic canals in a 51-year-old hypertensive male with sudden onset of visual loss in his left eye and an altitudinal inferior mainly temporal
visual field defect. Sequential axial sections (*a*) show luxury pneumatization
of the sphenoid sinus extending into the lesser wing of the sphenoid bone
and elevation of the bony optic canal. The carotid arteries cause deep groove
into the sphenoid sinus (upper left and right). The moderately ectatic left internal carotid artery reaches deep into the intracranial end of the optic canal
(lower right). Configuration of the narrowed and tortuous optic canals viewed
with a bone window (*b*): The extension of the sphenoid sinus backward reduces
the lumen of the optic canal and sella turcica. Parasagittal computer reformation (*c*) through the intracranial end of the left optic canal and internal carotid
artery: The lumen of the optic canal is filled mainly by the artery obviously
displacing the optic nerve upwards and nasally. Paraxial computer reformation
perpendicular to the left (*d*) and right (*e*) intracranial end of the optic canal.
The lumen of the optic canal is filled by the hyperdense soft tissue representing
the internal carotid artery. The computer reformation through the right canal
shows the normal low density

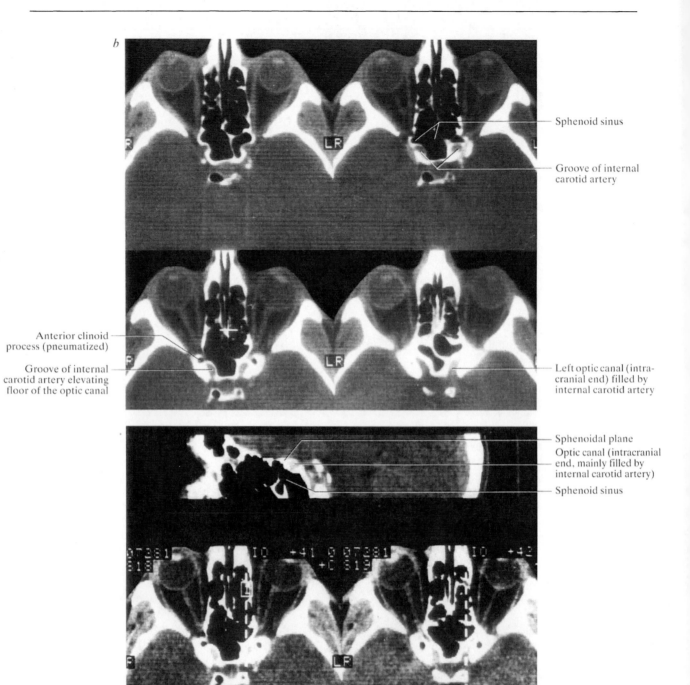

b

Sphenoid sinus

Groove of internal carotid artery

Anterior clinoid process (pneumatized)

Groove of internal carotid artery elevating floor of the optic canal

Left optic canal (intracranial end) filled by internal carotid artery

Sphenoidal plane

Optic canal (intracranial end, mainly filled by internal carotid artery)

Sphenoid sinus

c

Fig. 40b, c

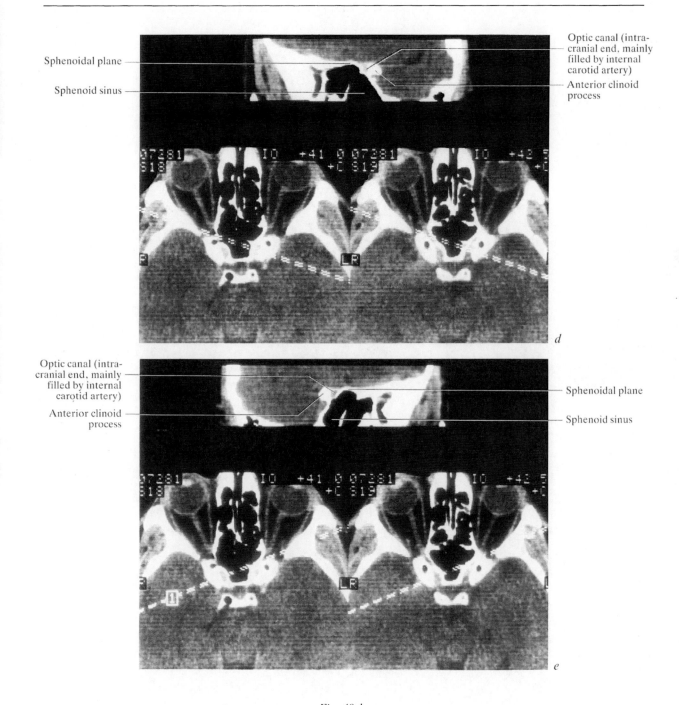

Sphenoidal plane

Sphenoid sinus

Optic canal (intra-cranial end, mainly filled by internal carotid artery)

Anterior clinoid process

d

Optic canal (intra-cranial end, mainly filled by internal carotid artery)

Anterior clinoid process

Sphenoidal plane

Sphenoid sinus

e

Fig. 40 d, e

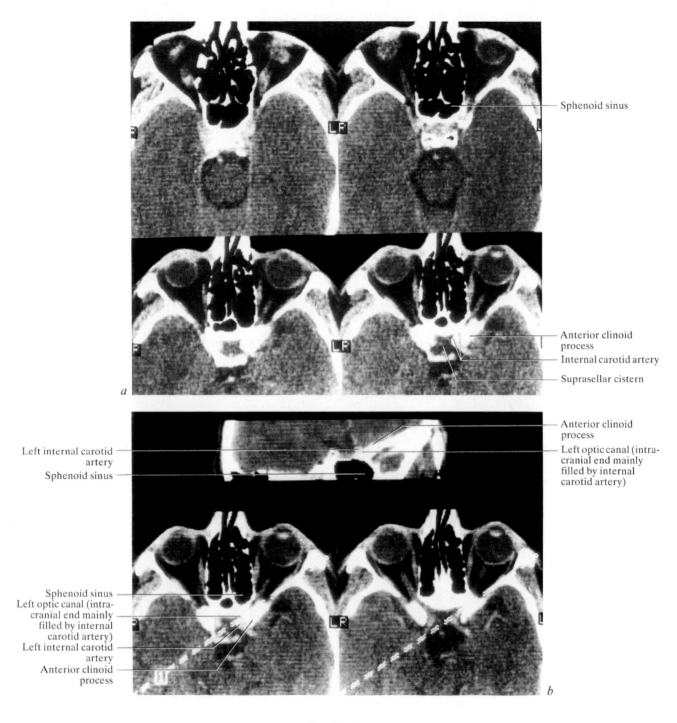

Sphenoid sinus

Anterior clinoid process

Internal carotid artery

Suprasellar cistern

Anterior clinoid process

Left optic canal (intra-cranial end mainly filled by internal carotid artery)

Left internal carotid artery

Sphenoid sinus

Sphenoid sinus

Left optic canal (intra-cranial end mainly filled by internal carotid artery)

Left internal carotid artery

Anterior clinoid process

Fig. 41 a, b

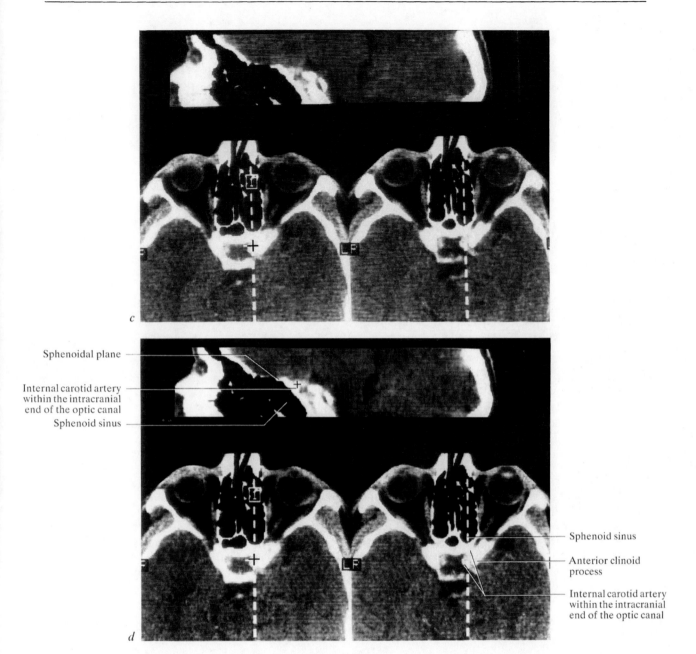

Sphenoidal plane

Internal carotid artery
within the intracranial
end of the optic canal

Sphenoid sinus

Sphenoid sinus

Anterior clinoid
process

Internal carotid artery
within the intracranial
end of the optic canal

Fig. 41a–d. Moderate dolichoectasia of the left internal carotid artery in a 50-year-old male with a superior altitudinal visual field defect and corresponding optic atrophy. Sequential axial CT sections (*a*) show a well pneumatized sphenoid sinus and a slightly narrowed steep optic canal, the intracranial end of which is almost filled by the moderately ectatic carotid artery (lower right). Paraxial computer reformations parallel to the intracranial end of the optic canal (*b*): The enlarged left internal carotid artery is visualized within the intracranial end of the optic canal, taking up most of its lumen. Parasagittal computer reformation through the intracranial end of the optic foramen (*c*) demonstrating the ectatic vessel occupying most of its lumen. In Fig. 41d the internal carotid artery is identified by a localizing marker (white cross), which has been placed right on the artery (lower left) proving that the hyperdense structure within the intracranial canal is the ectatic vessel (*d,* above)

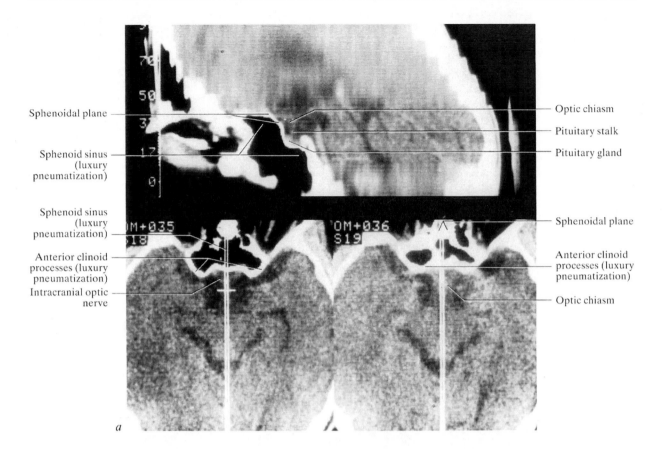

Sphenoidal plane

Sphenoid sinus
(luxury
pneumatization)

Sphenoid sinus
(luxury
pneumatization)

Anterior clinoid
processes (luxury
pneumatization)

Intracranial optic
nerve

Optic chiasm

Pituitary stalk

Pituitary gland

Sphenoidal plane

Anterior clinoid
processes (luxury
pneumatization)

Optic chiasm

Fig. 42a, b. Pneumosinus of the sphenoid sinus and lesser wing of the sphenoid bone in a 14-year-old boy with partial hemiatrophy and severe bilateral optic atrophy. (*a*) Sagittal computer reformation (above) and axial CT section through the extensively pneumatized anterior clinoid processes. Note massive pneumatization of the sphenoid sinus with elevation of the planum sphenoidale. (*b*) Coronal computer reformation (above) and axial CT sections through both optic canals. Due to excessive pneumatization of the sphenoid sinus and anterior clinoid processes there is significant narrowing of the slit-like optic canals (reversed image, bone dark, air white)

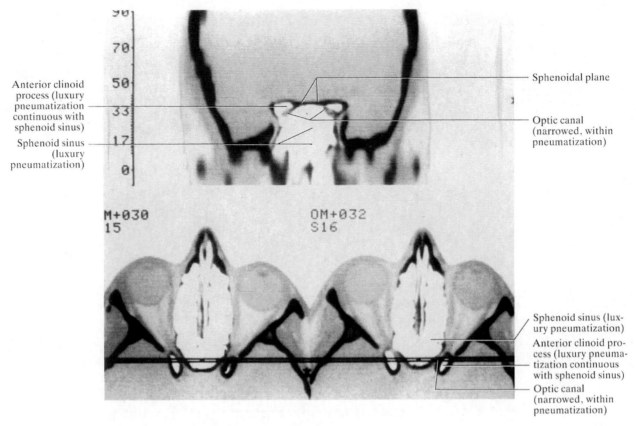

Anterior clinoid process (luxury pneumatization continuous with sphenoid sinus)

Sphenoid sinus (luxury pneumatization)

Sphenoidal plane

Optic canal (narrowed, within pneumatization)

Sphenoid sinus (luxury pneumatization)

Anterior clinoid process (luxury pneumatization continuous with sphenoid sinus)

Optic canal (narrowed, within pneumatization)

Fig. 42b

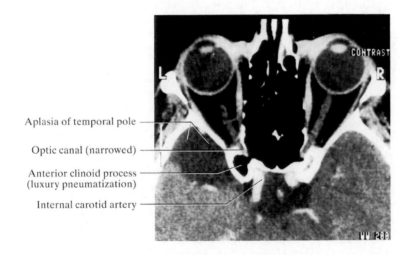

Aplasia of temporal pole

Optic canal (narrowed)

Anterior clinoid process (luxury pneumatization)

Internal carotid artery

Fig. 43. Pneumosinus dilatans in the vicinity of a low density area in front of the left temporal lobe (aplasia of temporal pole) in a 60-year-old female with progressive optic atrophy (Courtesy of Dr. Möller, Stade). There is considerable pneumatization of the anterior clinoid process with narrowing of the left optic foramen

67

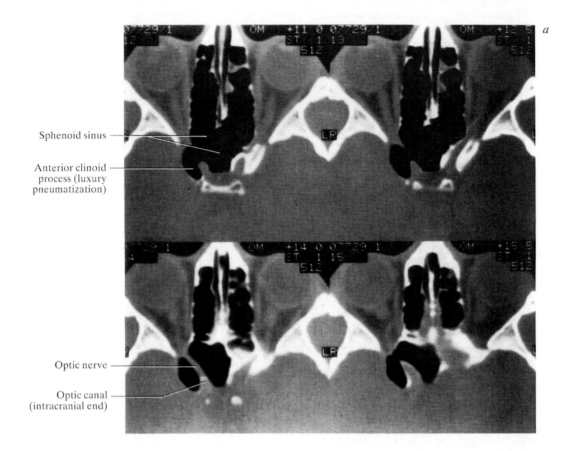

Sphenoid sinus

Anterior clinoid
process (luxury
pneumatization)

Optic nerve

Optic canal
(intracranial end)

a

Fig. 44a–c. Unilateral pneumosinus of the right sphenoid sinus and lesser wing
of the sphenoid bone in a 26-year-old male who had experienced an episode
of fluctuating visual loss and headaches, which subsided spontaneously. There
was a very slight afferent pupillary defect. After a brief period with signs of
optic nerve compression, further extension of the pneumatocele has obviously
led to spontaneous decompression. Sequential axial sections (*a*) show massive
hyperpneumatization around the right optic canal (bone window). The optic
nerve appears to run through the aerocele of the sphenoid sinus. (*b*) Midsagittal
computer reformation through the planum sphenoidale demonstrating massive
pneumatization and bone erosion of the planum sphenoidale. (*c*) Coronal computer reformation through the optic canal demonstrating the extent of the
pneumatocele and bone erosion

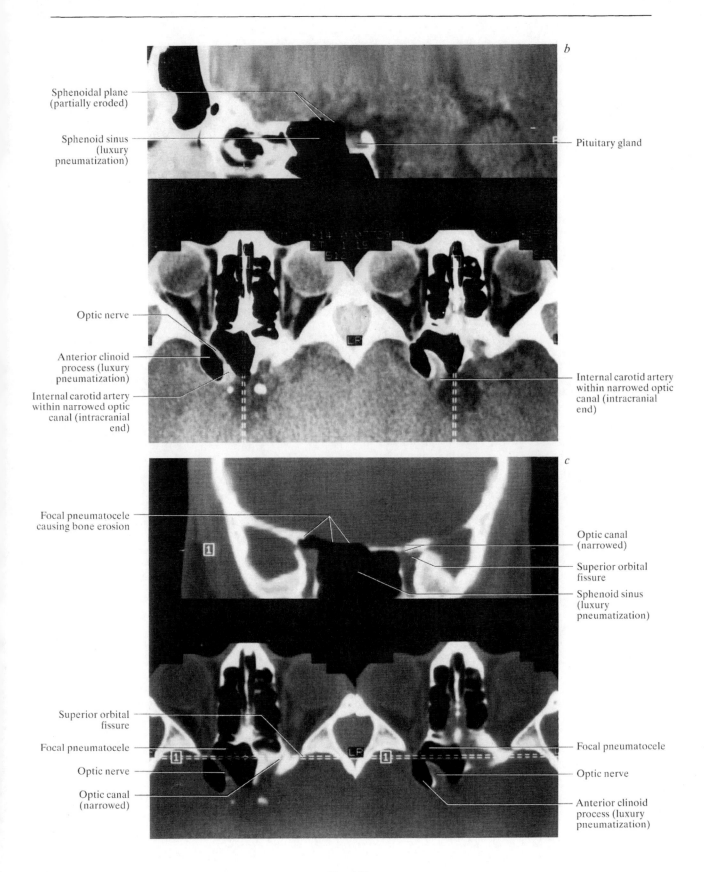

Sphenoidal plane (partially eroded)

Sphenoid sinus (luxury pneumatization)

Pituitary gland

Optic nerve

Anterior clinoid process (luxury pneumatization)

Internal carotid artery within narrowed optic canal (intracranial end)

Internal carotid artery within narrowed optic canal (intracranial end)

Focal pneumatocele causing bone erosion

Optic canal (narrowed)

Superior orbital fissure

Sphenoid sinus (luxury pneumatization)

Superior orbital fissure

Focal pneumatocele

Optic nerve

Optic canal (narrowed)

Focal pneumatocele

Optic nerve

Anterior clinoid process (luxury pneumatization)

Fig. 44 b, c

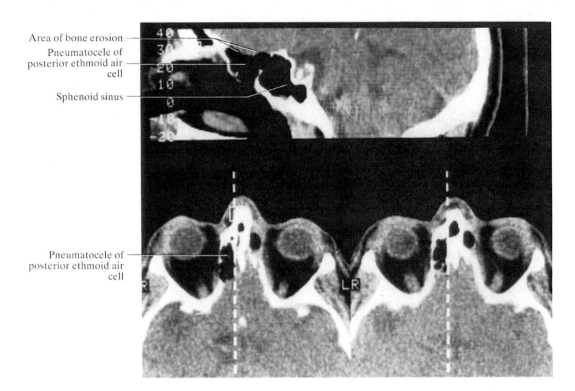

Area of bone erosion

Pneumatocele of posterior ethmoid air cell

Sphenoid sinus

Pneumatocele of posterior ethmoid air cell

Fig. 45. Excessive pneumatization of a posterior ethmoid air cell causing bone erosion of the planum sphenoidale in a 50-year-old male who experienced a CSF fistula during ethmoid surgery

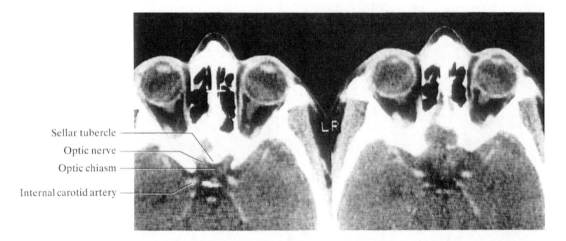

Sellar tubercle

Optic nerve

Optic chiasm

Internal carotid artery

Fig. 46. Prefixed chiasm in a 56-year-old woman with a central scotoma and slowly progressive optic atrophy. The optic chiasm, which is situated deep within the suprasellar cistern immediately behind and slightly below the level of the planum sphenoidale, is well visualized on axial sections through the intracranial end of the optic canals. Plane of section: about −10° to the orbital meatal baseline (see also Fig. 15)

70

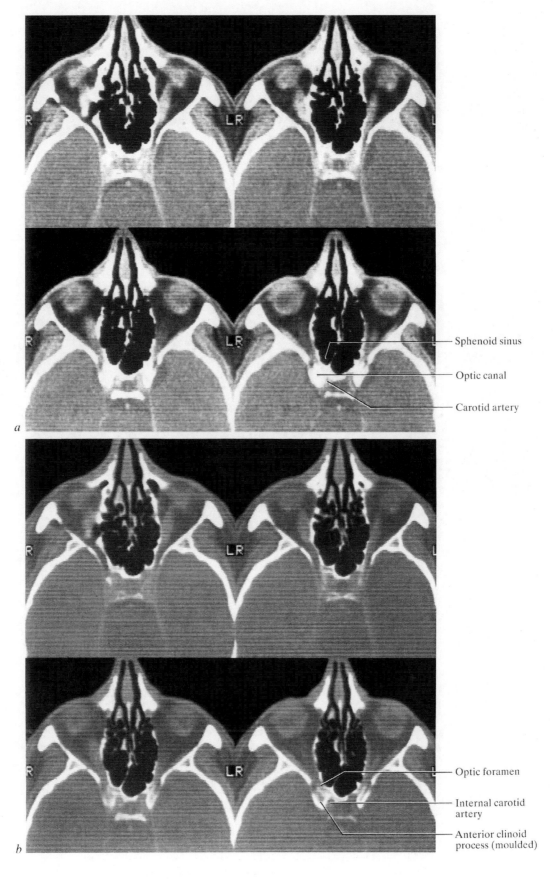

Sphenoid sinus

Optic canal

Carotid artery

Optic foramen

Internal carotid artery

Anterior clinoid process (moulded)

Fig. 47a, b. Legend see p. 72

71

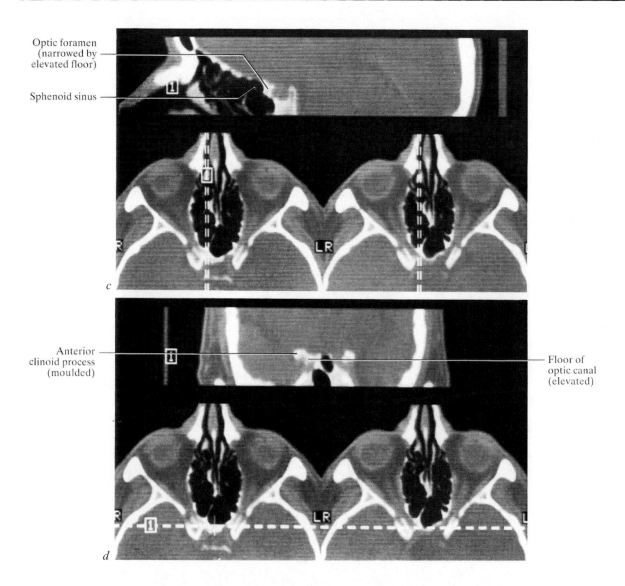

Optic foramen (narrowed by elevated floor)

Sphenoid sinus

Anterior clinoid process (moulded)

Floor of optic canal (elevated)

c

d

Fig. 47a–d. Axial CT-sections and parasagittal and coronal computer-reformations through the optic canals in a 58 year old hypertensive male with intermittent visual loss initially to 0.3 with a central and paracentral nasal scotoma, later on improvement of visual acuity to 1.0 in the presence of an almost complete loss of the nasal visual field and finally reduction of visual acuity to hand motion and a small residual island of the visual field in his right eye.

(*a*) Consecutive axial CT-sections through the optic canals viewed with a bone window (upper right lowest, lower left highest section): the anterior clinoid process of the right side appears enlarged and moulded at its posterior medial aspect by the internal carotid artery, which has elevated the floor of the right optic canal reducing its lumen and causing a characteristic double conture.

(*b*) Axial CT-section through the same plane viewed with a soft tissue window. The structure within the moulded right anterior clinoid process can be identified as the right internal carotid artery.

(*c*) Parasagittal computer reformation through the intracranial portion of the right optic canal (bone window): the elevated floor of the optic canal reduces the lumen and causes a double conture.

(*d*) Coronal computer reformation through the intracranial end of the optic canals (bone window): the moulded and enlarged right anterior clinoid process can be visualized as well as the elevation of the floor of the optic canal caused by chronic pressure of the right internal carotid artery

7
Pterional Approach for Microsurgical Decompression of the Optic Nerve

H.-R. EGGERT

The intracanalicular portion of the optic nerve can be approached by different ways, depending on the location of the lesion. Lesions located exclusively at the medial wall of the optic canal can be reached by a transethmoidal approach (Niho et al. 1970). The roof and the lateral wall may be inspected by a subfrontal or frontolateral extradural approach (Brihaye 1976; Housepian 1978; Schürmann et al. 1961). Only intradural approaches provide the possibility of examining the lateral and medial wall and the roof of the optic canal and the entire length of the optic nerve. Since intradural approaches involve the risk of brain damage, the intradural way to the optic canal should be as short as possible. These requirements are met by the pterional approach (Fig. 48). In contrast to the subfrontal intradural approach, the risk of brain damage due to brain retraction can be diminished using the pterional approach by opening the arachnoid of the Sylvian fissure (Hassler et al. 1985; Seeger 1986; Yasargil et al. 1975).

The patient is rested in a supine position with the head slightly elevated in order to reduce venous pressure. After turning the head approximately 45° to the opposite side and overstretching it by about 20° it is fixed by a Mayfield clamp. In this position, the frontal lobe will drop back from the orbital roof by itself, especially in elder patients with brain atrophy. In younger patients Mannitol may be used in order to reduce intracranial pressure. The skin is incised in a curved line just behind the hairline from the midline to a point in front of the tragus. The incision is directed down to the skull, cutting the temporal fascia and muscle parallel with its fibers (Fig. 49). After dissecting the temporal muscle from the temporal bone basally as far as possible and detaching it from the frontal part of the zygomatic arch, the skin-muscle flap is turned down in a basal direction. Thus, the laterobasal part of the frontal bone including the lateral orbital rim and the anterior part of temporal bone are exposed. Using three basal, one frontolateral and one tempo-

ral burr holes, a frontotemporal bone flap is removed. Basal
burr holes are situated just in front of and just behind the junc-
tion of the linea temporalis and lateral orbital rim and temporo-
basally. Using a high-speed drill, the lesser wing of the sphenoid
bone is removed down to the lateral edge of the superior orbital
fissure (Fig. 50). Additionally, temporal bone is removed basally.
In general, bone resection should extend basally as far as possible. Nevertheless, destruction of the orbital rim or opening of
the orbital cavity should be avoided.

The dura is opened in a curved incision over the basal frontal
lobe and the temporal pole and reflected basally. The arachnoid
of the Sylvian fissure is incised laterally in order to release cerebrospinal fluid. Opening of the Sylvian fissure is continued in
a medial direction down to the cistern of the carotid artery
(Fig. 51). The reason for opening the Sylvian fissure is to prevent
traction at the temporal lobe or superficial Sylvian veins when
the frontal lobe is elevated. Sacrifice of superficial Sylvian veins
should be avoided. In some cases medially located veins, drain-
ing the basal frontal lobe and crossing the medial part of the
Sylvian fissure have to be coagulated and divided in order to
prevent unintended tearing. Incision of the some-times rather
firm arachnoid may be facilitated when it is stretched by slight
elevation of the frontal lobe. However, strangulation of arteries
or veins due to stretching of the arachnoid has to be avoided.
Once the carotid cistern is opened, the frontal lobe is slightly
elevated using a self-retaining retractor and the arachnoid of
the optic cistern is opened from the carotid artery to the midline.
Adhesions between optic nerve and gyrus rectus and olfactory
nerve are dissected, treating all arteries feeding the optic nerve
extremely gently. Thus the intra-cisternal portion of the optic
nerve from the chiasm to its entrance into the optic canal is
exposed.

In order to open the optic canal, the dura overlying the
canal is incised along approximately 15 mm in the direction of
the canal. The rim of the dura fold covering the optic nerve
before its entrance into the osseous canal is spared 2–3 mm in
width at this stage of the procedure. Additional incisions are
made from the base of the anterior clinoid process parallel to
the dural fold in the direction of the planum sphenoidale and
parallel to this incision over the orbital roof. Thus, the frontoba-
sal dura above the optic canal can be reflected medially and
laterally like two wings of a door. On dissecting the dura above
the optic canal it should be borne in mind that the osseous
roof of the canal may be absent in some cases. These defects
are preferably located at the intracranial opening of the canal.

The roof of the canal is opened with a diamond drill of 4 mm diameter. In order to prevent overheating, only low speed and continuous irrigation is used. For resection of the lateral and medial wall a drill of 1 mm diameter is applied. In order to avoid undue pressure on the optic nerve, rongeurs are not used. The length of the artificial osseous defect should be extended to the orbital roof. Removing the medial and the lateral wall of the canal, mucosa of the sphenoid sinus or of a pneumatised anterior clinoid process can be exposed. Usually, the mucosa is left unopened. Nevertheless, in these cases the opening of paranasal sinuses should be closed, for instance by a transplant of subcutaneous fat tissue glued into the defect with fibrin sealant. After removing the roof and widening the medial and lateral wall of the optic canal, the dural fold and the dural sheath of the optic nerve can be opened. Under high magnification, the middle third of the dural sheath is elevated with sharp hook and incised longitudinally in the direction of the dural fold. Then, the dural fold is completely cut and the distal part of the dural sheath is opened up to the anulus Zinnii. This order of technical steps is applied in order to avoid any pressure on the optic nerve, which is most likely at the edge of the dural fold. Finally, adhesions between the nerve and the dural sheath, which are most common within the middle third of its intracanalicular course, are detached by sharp dissection (Fig. 52). Active hemostasis is usually not necessary. It has to be avoided at the optic nerve itself. The defect of the optic canal can be covered with fat tissue or a collagene pad which is fixed by fibrin glue. After filling up the subdural cavity with Ringer's solution, the dura is closed as tight as possible. The bone flap is replaced and fixed by sutures in at least three places. Burr holes and basal osseous defects may be filled with bone meal derived from drilling the burr holes. A suction drainage is inserted and left in place for 2 days. After suturing the temporal fascia and the galea, the skin is closed.

This approach will present no great difficulties to any surgeon who is experienced in microneurosurgery. Taking into account the precautions mentioned above it is safe for the patient, and additional trauma to the optic nerve is extremely unlikely. Prognosis for visual function depends usually primarily on the degree of preoperative optic atrophy.

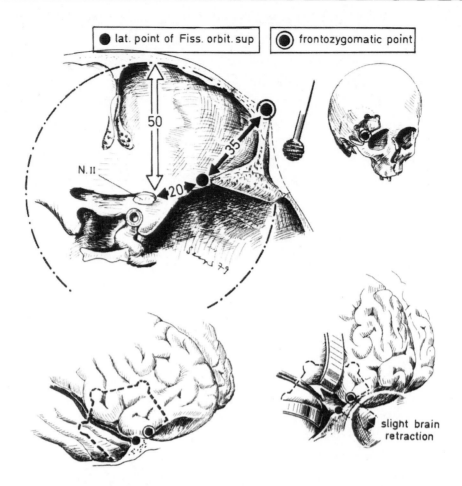

Fig. 48. Principles of the pterional approach to the intracranial and intracanalicular portion of the optic nerve. (From Seeger 1980, with kind permission of the author)

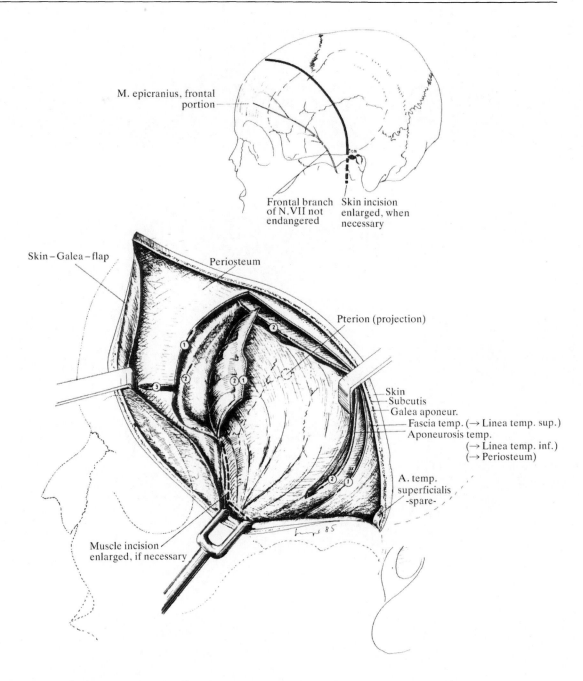

Fig. 49. Skin incision and detachment of temporal muscle for the pterional approach. Numbers in circles correspond to the order of surgical steps. (From Seeger 1986, with kind permission of the author)

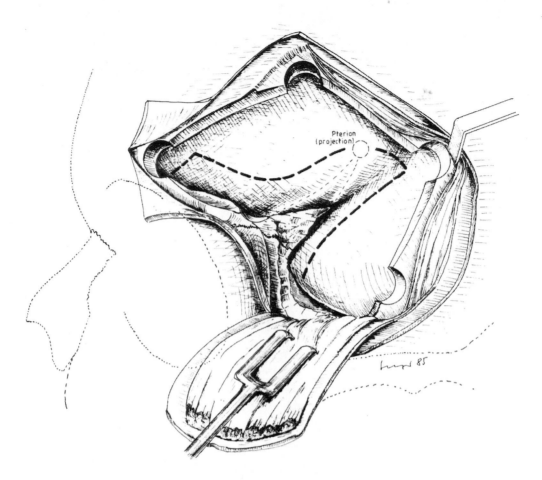

Fig. 50. Trepanation. The free bone flap is stored in a disinfectant. (From Seeger 1986, with kind permission of the author)

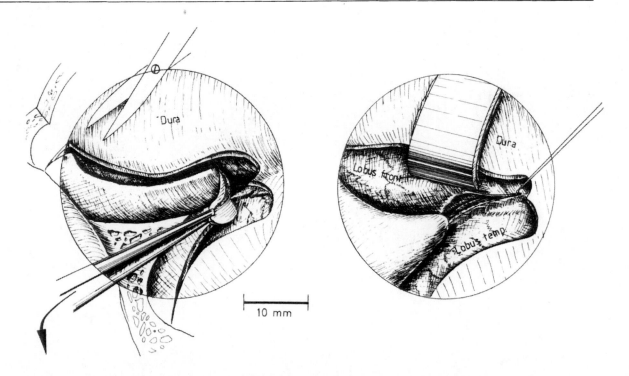

Fig. 51. Dural incision and opening of the Sylvian fissure. (From Seeger 1986, with kind permission of the author)

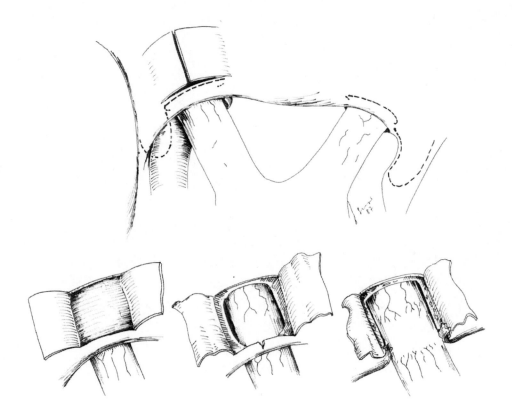

Fig. 52. Steps of unroofing the intracanalicular portion of the optic nerve

79

8
Intraoperative Findings in Patients with Intracanalicular Optic Nerve Compression

H.-R. Eggert

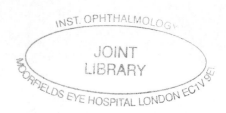
INST. OPHTHALMOLOGY
JOINT
LIBRARY
MOORFIELDS EYE HOSPITAL LONDON EC1V 9EL

We review the intraoperative findings in seven patients, who underwent microsurgical decompression of the optic nerve. In two cases the left and in five patients the right optic nerve were decompressed.

Various findings observed during surgical decompression of the optic nerve, the pathological significance of which remains doubtful. Especially, if an extradural approach is used for un-roofing the optic canal, most unequivocal signs of optic nerve compression will probably be overlooked. These can only be recognized using an intradural approach since they are mainly located at the intracranial opening of the optic canal including the dural fold forming the roof of the intracranial opening of the optic canal. Pathologic conditions of the optic nerve and surrounding structures may be observed during surgery at the intracranial portion of the nerve as well as at its intracanalicular part and at the walls of the osseous optic canal.

In three of seven patients who underwent microsurgical decompression of the optic nerve, more or less strong adhesions between gyrus rectus, olfactory nerve and the intracisternal segment of the optic nerve were found. However, it seemed unlikely that these adhesions contributed significantly to the syndrome of optic nerve compression.

Flattening of the optic nerve was observed in four patients 2–3 mm before its intracranial entrance under the covering dural fold. In each of these cases, the nerve was bulging upward, being strangled by the rim of the dural fold. Bulging was caused by the underlying internal carotid artery in one case and by the ophthalmic artery in the other (Fig. 53). Due to the anatomical relationships in the other two cases it was not possible to discern which artery caused the bulging.

Superficial vascularization of the optic nerve appeared inconspicuous in one of these four patients. In a second patient it seemed rarefied. In the other two cases, there was a distinct hypervascularization of the optic nerve 2–3 mm before it entered the canal, possibly representing neovascularization. Additionally, there was a pneumosinus dilatans of the sphenoid sinus in one of these four patients.

Atrophy of the intracisternal segment of the optic nerve was observed in two patients with a nerve diameter of less than 3 mm. One of these cases had a bilateral pneumosinus dilatans of the sphenoid sinus with pneumatization of the anterior clinoid process. In this case, atrophy of both optic nerves was observed. In the other patient, only the decompressed nerve showed atrophy along its entire course from the chiasm to the annulus of Zinn. The contralateral optic nerve appeared inconspicuous as far as its intracisternal segment was concerned. However, the atrophic nerve showed a discolored pale area at its dorsomedial circumference just underneath the intracranial opening of the osseous optic canal. Additionally, there was lack of superficial vascularization of the nerve within its intracanalicular portion. These observations might be interpreted as the final stage of a chronic compression syndrome.

The intracanalicular segment of the optic nerve became accessible during operation in five of seven patients. In two cases the dural sheath of the nerve was not opened. In one of these, there were strong arachnoid adhesions between the nerve and the dural sheath and the surgeon decided not to open the sheath in order to avoid traumatization of the nerve. In the other patient, a primarily extradural approach was used. Of the remaining five patients, the intracanalicular part of the nerve appeared inconspicuous in two. In one patient there were also strong arachnoidal adhesions between the nerve and its dural sheath. After osseous decompression, opening of the sheath and detachment of the adhesions, the nerve bulged into the artificial osseous defect. In the remaining two patients, the nerve showed a *pale discolored area* at its dorsomedial circumference underneath its entrance into the osseous optic canal. In one of these cases, the nerve was atrophied over its whole length as described before. In the other patient, superficial vessels were narrowed within the area of the pale spot (Fig. 54c, d).

Pressure erosion of the osseous optic canal was observed in three patients. In one of them with a pneumosinus dilatans of the sphenoid sinus, medial and basal parts of the wall were absent, thus providing a direct contact between the mucosa of the sphenoid sinus und the dural sheath of the optic nerve. The other two cases showed defects of the osseous roof of the optic canal near the region of its intracranial entrance. In one of these patients, the roof was partially absent, showing a V-shaped defect of 4 mm length. In the other patient, the elliptic defect left the rim of the osseous roof intact and was located within the middle third of the canal. However, underneath this elliptic osseous defect the optic nerve showed a pale area of the same size with narrowed superficial vessels as described before (Fig. 54a, b).

Some of the peculiarities observed during microsurgical decompression of the optic nerve may be due to variations of normal conditions. For instance, thinning of the osseous roof of the optic canal in the region of its intracranial opening as well as osseous defects of this part are also observed in healthy subjects as sequelae of the normal aging process (Lang 1981). However, if the segment of the optic nerve underlying such a defect appears discolored and lacks normal vascularization, in our opinion these findings should rather be interpreted as sequels of chronic compression. More obvious signs of optic nerve compression are flattening and bulging of the nerve with simultaneous strangulation at the edge of the dural fold covering the intracranial opening of the optic canal. In these cases, the nerve is forced to bulge out by the underlying internal carotid or ophthalmic artery. Thus the nerve is compressed between these vessels at its basolateral aspect and the dural fold or the osseous optic canal at its dorsomedial site. Using this criteria, unequivocal signs of optic nerve compression have been observed in five of seven patients. In one patient complete assessment was not possible due to a primarily extradural approach. In the remaining case the optic nerve was atrophic but showed a discolored area at its dorsomedial aspect, which might also have been the result of chronic nerve compression.

Table 1. Summary of findings in microsurgical decompression of the intracanalicular optic nerve

	B.,E. f 66 y left	C.,G. f 45 y right	D.,M. f 43 y right	G.,C. f 52 y right	K.,G. m 44 y left	S.,E. m 55 y right	W.,J. m 43 y right
Intracranial optic nerve							
flattened	+	−	−	+	+	+	−
strangled	+	−	−	+	+	+	−
bulging	+	−	−	+	+	+	−
hypervascularization	−	−	−	−	+	+	−
hypovascularization	−	+	−	−	−	−	−
arachnoid adhesions	−	−	+	+	−	−	+
atrophy	−	+	+	−	−	−	−
Intracanalicular optic nerve							
arachnoid adhesions	+	−	−	−	+	−	−
hypovascularization	−	+	−	−	−	−	+
pale area	−	+	−	−	−	−	+
bulging after decompression	+	−	−	−	−	−	−
atrophy	−	+	−	−	−	−	−
inconspicuous	−	−	−	+	−	+	−
unknown	−	−	+	−	−	−	−
Osseous optic canal							
defect of med. and basal wall	−	−	−	−	+	−	−
defect of roof	−	−	−	−	−	+	+
pneumosinus	−	−	+	−	+	−	−
inconspicuous	+	+	−	+	−	−	−

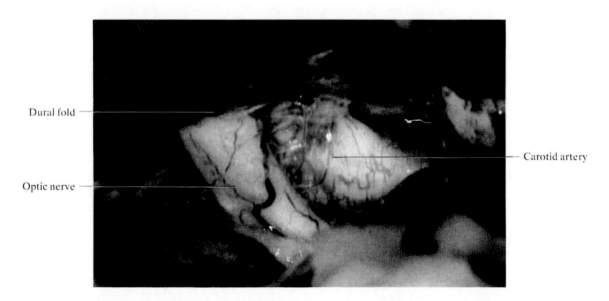

Dural fold

Optic nerve

Carotid artery

Fig. 53. Compression of the right optic nerve at the dural fold by the dolichoectatic internal carotid artery. (Case 1 of selected case reports)

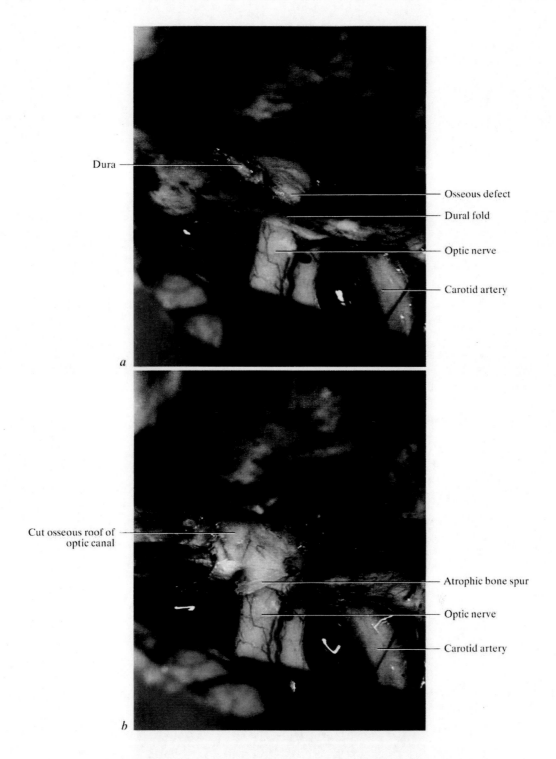

Dura

Osseous defect
Dural fold
Optic nerve
Carotid artery

a

Cut osseous roof of
optic canal

Atrophic bone spur
Optic nerve
Carotid artery

b

Fig. 54. (*a*) Intracisternal portion of the right optic nerve, the dura over the roof of the optic canal has been partially detached displaying an elliptic osseous defect of the roof. (Case 3 of selected reports). (*b*) Following complete dissection of the dural fold convering the optic nerve an atrophic bone spur is removed

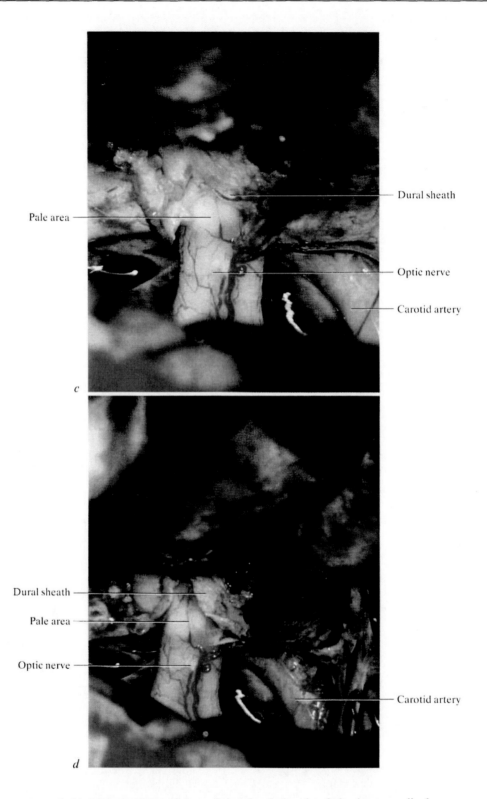

Pale area —

— Dural sheath

— Optic nerve

— Carotid artery

c

Dural sheath —

Pale area —

Optic nerve —

— Carotid artery

d

Fig. 54. (*c*) After partial opening of the dural sheath of the intracanalicular optic nerve a pale area with narrowed superficial vessels is observed underneath the elliptic osseous defect. (*d*) Complete opening of the dural sheath, the most distal portion of the optic nerve is not visualized. Superficial vessels narrowed within the area of the pale spot gain normal width beyond the lesion

86

9

Selected Case Reports

R. Unsöld

Case I (G. CH. 201234)

*Compression of the right optic nerve
by a dolichoectatic carotid artery*

A 52-year-old female had her last ophthalmological examination
in October 1985. At that time visual acuity was in both eyes 1.2.
Both optic nerve heads were well defined, there was no optic
atrophy. In Juli 1986 she saw a "shadow" in front of her right
eye and recognized reduction of visual acuity. An ophthalmological examination on September 9, 1986 revealed a superior altitudinal visual field defect, reduction of visual acuity in the right
eye to 0.2 and a central and paracentral superior altitudinal scotoma. The left eye had a visual acuity of 1.2 and a normal visual
field. Reexamination on September 14, 1986 showed further reduction of visual acuity of the right eye to 0.1 and later to 0.04.
At that time there was, in addition to the central scotoma,
marked constriction of the visual field. CT was performed and
showed the right internal carotid artery reaching deep into the
right optic foramen, probably compressing the right optic nerve,
which was visualized as a slit-like area of low density within
the optic canal (Fig. 57). On October 27, 1986 the patient underwent decompressive surgery by a pterional approach. During
surgery considerable dolichoectasia of the internal carotid artery
was observed, and the right optic nerve was elevated by the
ectatic vessel at the intracranial end of the optic foramen. There
were slight arachnoid adhesions around the optic nerve. The
following day there was a significant increase of visual acuity
of the right eye to 0.5, the peripheral visual field appeared to
be restored in all directions. In a postoperative examination
about one week after surgery, visual acuity had increased to
0.6 p–0.8 p. The visual field showed, apart from the remaining
small, mainly paracentral scotoma, almost complete restitution

(Fig. 61). Comparison of the preoperative and postoperative VER (Fig. 56) failed to reflect an electrophysiologic correlated despite the impressive improvement of visual acuity and visual field.

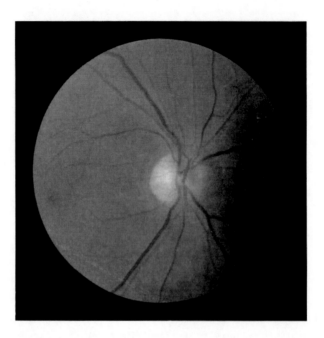

Fig. 55. Funduscopic appearance of the right optic disk prior to surgery. There is significant atrophy of the optic nerve head

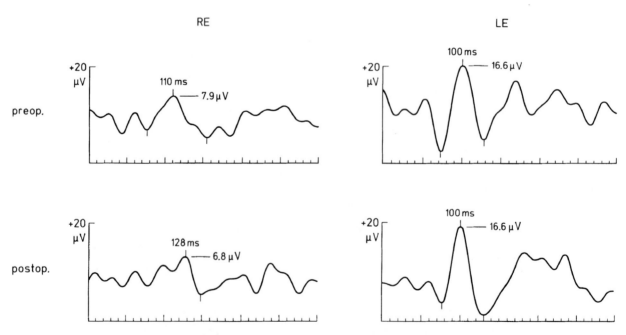

Fig. 56. Pre- and postoperative VEP of Case 1. There is no significant change after decompression despite the impressive improvement of visual acuity and visual field (see also Fig. 26)

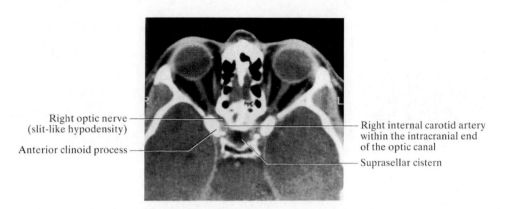

Right optic nerve —
(slit-like hypodensity)

Anterior clinoid process —

— Right internal carotid artery
within the intracranial end
of the optic canal

— Suprasellar cistern

Fig. 57. Axial CT section through the optic canal in a plane of section of about −10° to the orbito-meatal base line. Both optic canals are visualized. On both sides the intracranial end of the optic canal is filled by a structure of higher density than the optic nerve representing the internal carotid artery, which shows some calcification of its wall in its supraclinoid portion. On the right side the posterior half of the optic canal is filled by the internal carotid artery, obviously compressing the optic nerve, which can be seen as a slit-like area of lower density within the optic canal. On the left side the intracanalicular section of the optic nerve is considerably larger and appears as an oval structure of lower density

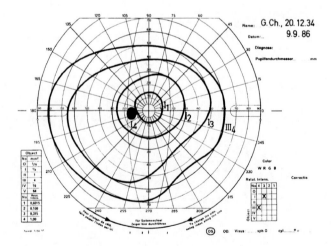

Fig. 58. Left visual field showing normal isopters

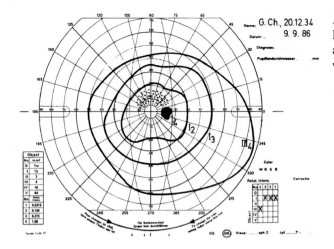

Fig. 59. Visual field of the right eye at the onset of visual loss: besides the central scotoma there is a paracentral altitudinal superior scotoma. Visual acuity at that time was 0.2

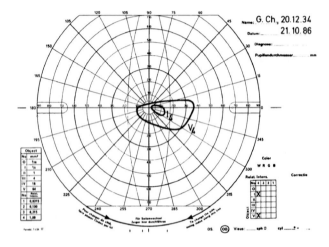

Fig. 60. Visual field immediately before surgery: there is marked constriction of the entire visual field as well as a central scotoma. Visual acuity was at that time 0.04

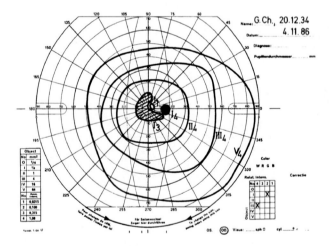

Fig. 61. Visual field of the right eye about one week after surgery: there is significant restitution of the peripheral visual field with almost normal isopters, and a rather large paracentral residual scotoma corresponding to the preoperatively visible optic atrophy of the right nerve head. Visual acuity was at that time 0.6–0.8 p

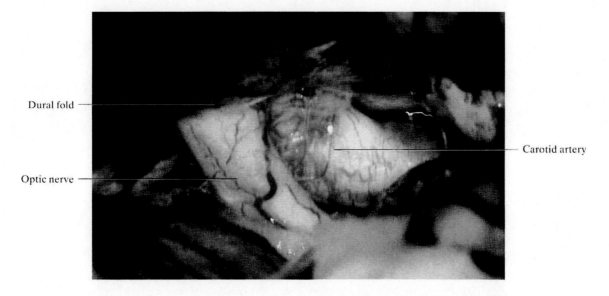

Dural fold

Optic nerve

Carotid artery

Fig. 62. Surgical photography of case 1. There is compression of the right optic nerve at the dural fold by the dolichoectatic internal carotid artery

Summary

A 52-year-old woman showed progressive visual loss starting with an altitudinal superior and central scotoma and slowly progressive optic atrophy. Visual acuity dropped to 0.04, there was marked constriction of the right visual field. During surgery an ectatic carotid artery was seen to compress the right optic nerve within the optic canal. Immediately after surgery there was marked improvement of visual acuity. About one week after surgery visual acuity increased from 0.04 to 0.6 p–0.8 p and impressive restitution of the visual field occurred.

Bilateral optic nerve compression by a slightly dolichoectatic carotid artery in the presence of narrowing of both optic foramina due to hyperpneumatization of the sphenoid sinus and a left pneumosinus dilatans of the lesser wing of the sphenoid bone

A 55-year-old male observed after an upper respiratory infection for the first time a "shadow" in front of his left eye, which resolved spontaneously. When he was first examined on May 3, 1985 visual acuity in the right eye was 0.25, in the left 1.2. There was a slight left afferent pupillary defect, but no significant color desaturation. The visual field of the right eye was normal, the visual field of the left eye showed constriction of the lower nasal quadrant (Fig. 65a). There was moderate but significant optic atrophy in the left eye (Fig. 63b). Reexamination on the May 22 revealed slight progression of visual loss to 0.9 and further constriction of the inferior nasal quadrant of the left visual field, as well as a slight paracentral scotoma (Fig. 65c). A computerized tomogram was performed, which showed narrowing of both optic canals due to hyperpneumatization of the sphenoid sinus and pneumosinus dilatans reaching from the sphenoid sinus continuously into the left anterior clinoid process with the suspicion of optic nerve compression against the slightly enlarged internal carotid artery reaching into the intracranial end of the left optic canal. The diagnosis of suspected optic nerve compression in the presence of a left pneumosinus dilatans was made and decompressive surgery was recommended in the case of further deterioration. On September 22 the patient returned because of rapidly progressive visual loss in his right eye associated with pain projected in his right orbit and hypaesthesia and dysaesthesia in the supply area of the first and second branch of the right trigeminal nerve. At that time visual acuity in the right eye was reduced to 0.5 and in the left eye to 0.8, but was reported to be fluctuating in both eyes. The right visual field showed besides a central scotoma a mainly inferior altitudinal scotoma and marked constriction of the remaining upper half of the visual field (Fig. 65f). Color vision was significantly disturbed in the right eye and there was a marked right afferent pupillary defect. VEP examination showed marked reduction of amplitude and increased latency (Fig. 67). Acute right and chronic left optic nerve compression was suspected and the patient underwent decompressive surgery of the right optic nerve by a pterional approach on October 7, 1986. At surgery bone erosion over a distance of about 3 mm was detected within the roof of the optic canal, probably representing a sign of chronic compression. There was moderately increased vascularity of the optic nerve behind its entrance into the intracranial end of the optic foramen. The postoperative course was complicated by wound infection which required removal of the bone plasty but was successfully treated with antibiotics. There was a slight postoperative increase of visual acuity to 0.63 p–0.7 p in the right eye, but marked further visual loss had occurred in the left eye with a visual acuity of 0.5–0.63. The right visual field did not show significant improvement, on repeated examination the results of visual field examinations could not be well reproduced and the patient complained of fluctuating visual acuity. The visual field of the left eye showed an almost complete inferior altitudinal defect and constriction of the remaining upper half of the visual field. There was marked reduction of color perception in the left eye, previously not observed, and a marked afferent left pupillary defect. Ophthalmoscopy showed a slight increase of optic atrophy in both eyes. The patient refused decompressive surgery of the left optic nerve. On reexamination on February 17, 1987 visual acuity was 0.7–0.8 p in both eyes. There was still a marked left afferent pupillary defect and color dissaturation. The right visual field showed considerable improvement (Fig. 65g). VEP of the right eye (side of surgical decompression) showed improvement with still increased latency but an almost normal amplitude (Fig. 67). The patient was reluctant to undergo surgery, but will return for surgery when visual function further decreases in his left eye.

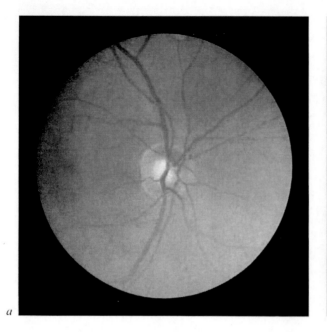
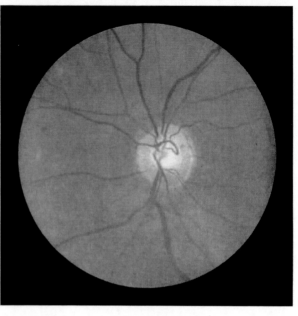

Fig. 63a, b. Photographs of both optic disks in Case 2 at the time of the first examination in May 1985. There is a normal optic disk in the right eye (*a*) and significant optic atrophy with some degree of cupping in the left eye (*b*)

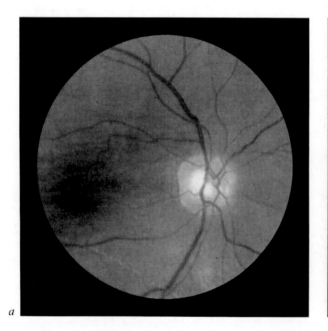
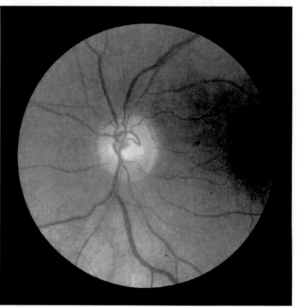

Fig. 64a, b. Photographs of both optic disks about two months after decompressive surgery of the right optic nerve. There is moderate atrophy of the right disk (*a*) and slightly increased atrophy of the left disk (*b*)

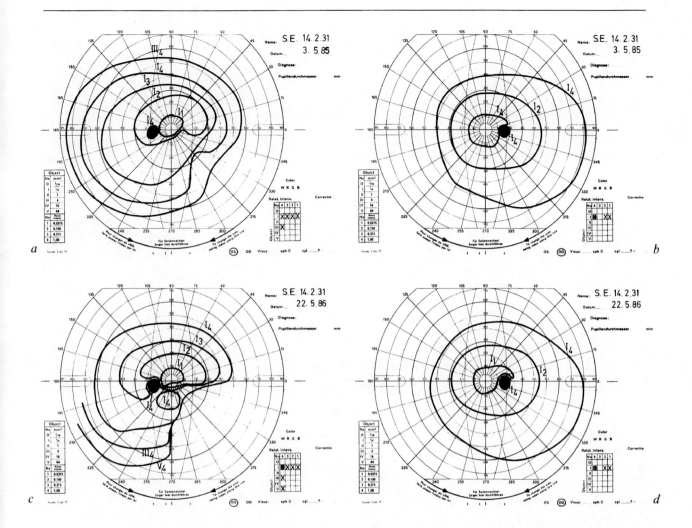

Fig. 65a–j. Visual field findings in Case 2 during the course of the disease (for details see discription of the case history). The right eye showed rapidly progressive visual field constriction with an central scotoma and inferior altitudinal defect, which improved considerably after decompressive surgery of the right optic nerve. The left eye showed first a chronic progressive inferior and later a complete inferior altitudinal defect with constriction of the remaining upper visual field. The findings remained fairly constant in the last three examinations

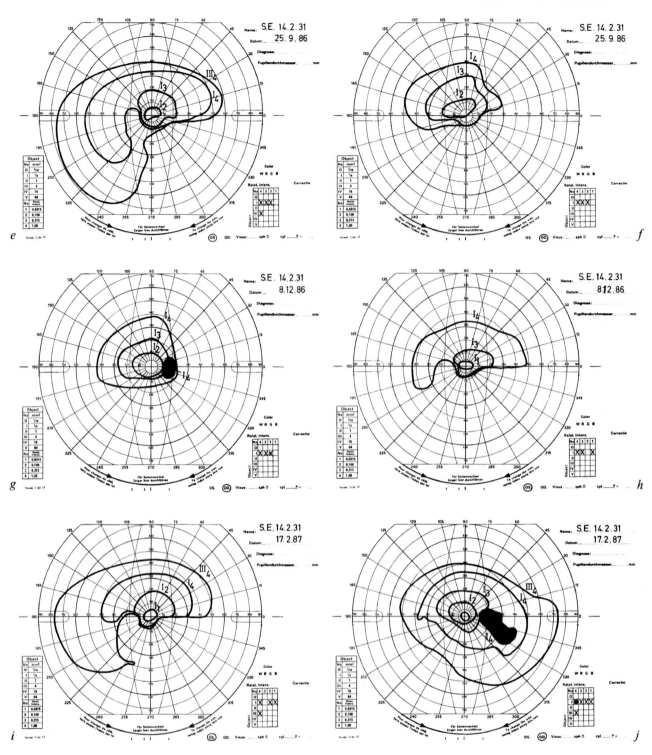

Fig. 65 e–j

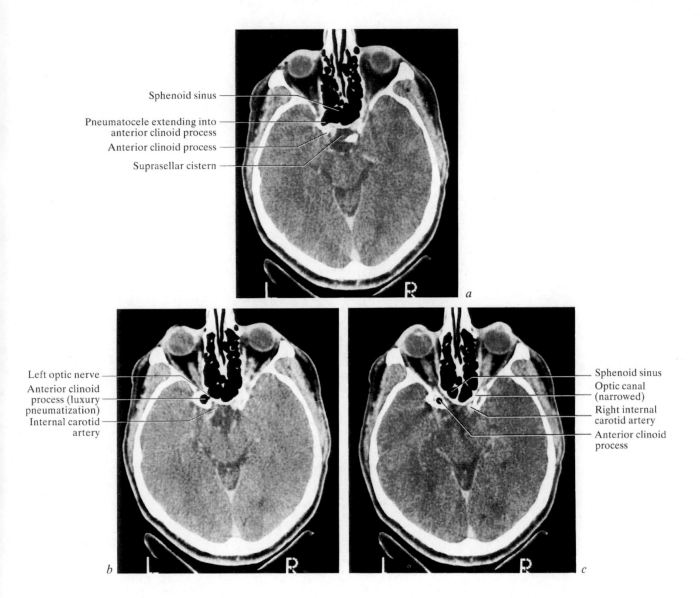

Sphenoid sinus

Pneumatocele extending into
anterior clinoid process

Anterior clinoid process

Suprasellar cistern

a

Left optic nerve

Anterior clinoid
process (luxury
pneumatization)

Internal carotid
artery

Sphenoid sinus

Optic canal
(narrowed)

Right internal
carotid artery

Anterior clinoid
process

b

c

Fig. 66 a–c. Sequential axial CT sections through the optic canal in Case 2 immediately before decompressive surgery of the right optic nerve. There is considerable pneumatization of the sphenoid sinus with bilateral narrowing of the optic
canal. The left anterior clinoid process shows continuous pneumatization from
the sphenoid sinus into the anterior clinoid process and suspicion of optic
nerve compression against the internal carotid artery at the intracranial optic
canal. The right internal carotid artery reaches deep into the intracranial opening of the narrowed right optic foramen. Both optic nerves' shadows appear
significantly enlarged, probably due to chronic congestion

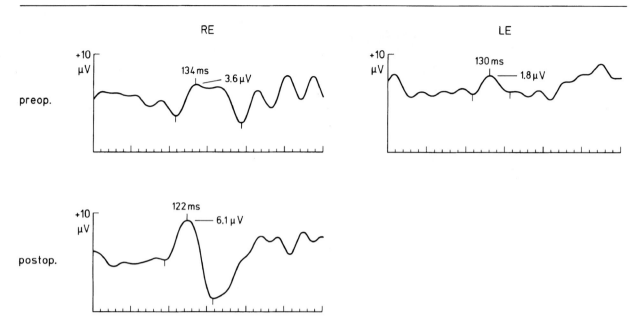

Fig. 67. Preoperative VEP findings in the right and left eye in Case 2 (above). The low amplitude combined with moderate latency increase points to blockage of conduction by compression. The postoperative increase of amplitude correlates with the functional improvement (below)

Summary

A 55-year-old male presented visual loss of the left eye and a lower nasal visual field defect, slight atrophy of the optic disk and other clinical signs of optic nerve compression. Visual failure was slowly progressive to a total inferior altitudinal scotoma with fluctuating visual acuity. CT showed narrowing of both optic canals due to marked pneumatization of the sphenoid sinus and the presence of a left pneumosinus dilatans of the lesser wing of the sphenoid bone. While the clinical signs were observed acute visual failure developed in the right eye with the clinical signs of optic nerve compression. The compressive mechanism by a dolichoectatic internal carotid artery could be verified at surgery. The postsurgical course was complicated by a wound infection, but there was significant postoperative improvement of visual function in the right eye. Decompressive surgery of the left optic nerve is planned when there is further progress of visual loss.

Case 3 (W. J. 210543)

Optic nerve compression by a dolichoectatic carotid artery within the right optic foramen

A 41-year-old hypertensive male in otherwise good health observed progressive visual loss in his right eye in spring 1984. The first ophthalmological examination revealed reduction of visual acuity in the right eye to 0.3 and a visual acuity of 1.0 p in the left eye. Besides a central scotoma there was a temporal visual field defect in the right eye (Fig. 69a). A diagnosis of optic neuritis was suspected and the patient was treated with steroids elsewhere. There was a slight improvement of the previously fluctuating visual acuity to 0.7 and a questionable improvement of the visual field. In December 1985 visual acuity in the left eye dropped to 0.8 p. Reexamination in April 1986 revealed a visual acuity of 0.3 in the right and of 0.6–0.8 in the left eye. There was a right afferent pupillary defect and significant optic atrophy of the right optic disk (Fig. 68a). The VER showed massive destruction of the potential with reduction of amplitude and increased latency, more marked in the right than the left eye. Thin section computerized tomography was performed and revealed increased soft tissue density within the right suprasellar cistern. There was slight molding of the medial aspect of the anterior clinoid process, elevation of the floor of the optic canal and an enlarged right internal carotid artery reaching deep into the intracranial end of the optic canal. The left internal carotid artery also reached into the left optic canal (Fig. 70). Cisternography did not show evidence of a soft tissue mass other than the carotid artery. The diagnosis of optic nerve compression was made and the patient underwent surgical decompression of the optic nerve. At surgery bone erosion of the roof of the optic canal was observed over an area of about 1 cm^2. The optic nerve within the optic foramen appeared constricted and whitish over a length of about 4 mm, a finding leading to a suspicion of ischemia due to local compression (Fig. 71a–d). In addition, the supplying vessels of the optic nerve in this area appeared narrowed but were of normal caliber or slightly congested proximal and distal of this area. There was an uneventful postoperative course. Five days after surgery, visual acuity in the right eye had improved from 0.3 to 0.4–0.5 p. The computed visual field examination showed significant improvement of the temporal scotoma (Fig. 69c). Postoperative VEP showed considerable increase of amplitude (Fig. 25). The postoperative findings remained stable over the next six months. Left optic nerve decompression is planned when progressive visual loss occurs.

Summary

A 41-year-old hypertensive male developed first fluctuating and later progressive visual loss in the right eye. Clinical findings and CT signs indicated optic nerve compression at the optic foramen, possibly by an enlarged internal carotid artery. The compressive mechanism was verified during decompressive surgery. Postoperatively there was moderate but significant improvement of visual function in the right eye according to the degree of preexisting optic atrophy.

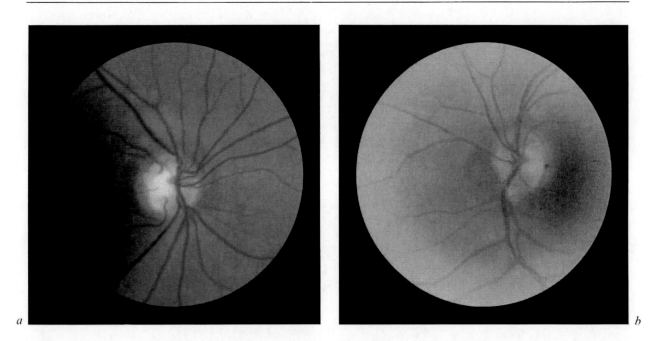

Fig. 68a, b. Fundusphotographs of both optic disks in Case 3. There is marked optic atrophy in the right eye (*a*) and a normal-appearing optic disk in the left eye (*b*)

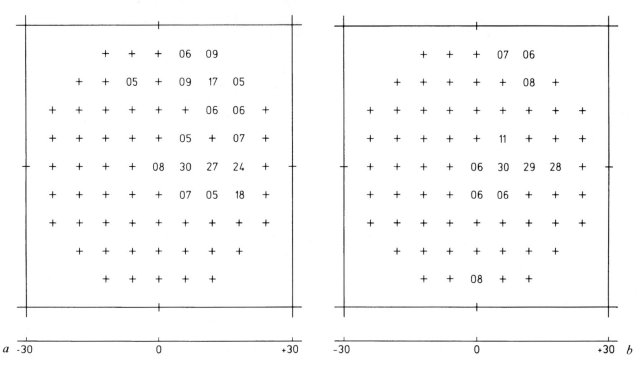

Fig. 69a, b. Computed perimetry of the right eye before (*a*) and after (*b*) surgery (Octopus, program 31). There is significant improvement of the temporal scotoma

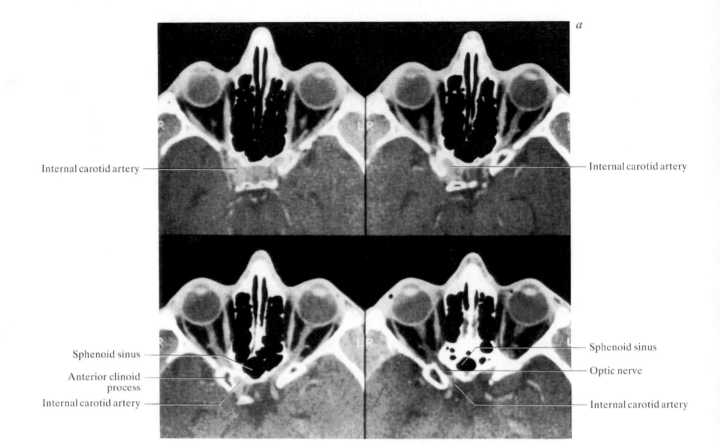

Internal carotid artery

Internal carotid artery

Sphenoid sinus

Sphenoid sinus

Anterior clinoid process

Optic nerve

Internal carotid artery

Internal carotid artery

a

Fig. 70. (*a*) Sequential axial CT sections through the optic canals (upper left lowest, lower right highest section). The sphenoid sinus appears well pneumatized. There is increased soft tissue density within the right suprasellar cistern and moderate enlargement of the right internal carotid artery, which extends into the optic canal. The right anterior clinoid process appears slightly molded and the medial wall of the optic canal appears elevated and shows a doublicated bony contour. The left internal carotid artery also extends into the intracranial opening of the optic canal. (*b*) Axial CT section through the chiasm. The chiasm lies close to the tuberculum sellae, the intracranial optic nerves are short, indicating a "prefixed chiasm". (*c*) Coronal computer reformation through the intracranial end of the optic foramen (plane of section indicated on axial CT section below). The lumen of the intracranial end of the optic canal is obturated by soft tissue density. Beneath the anterior clinoid process a roundish structure represents a cross section through the enlarged internal carotid artery, the supraclinoid portion of which fills the space of the intracranial opening of the optic foramen almost completely. The left internal carotid artery does not appear significantly enlarged but reaches deep into the intracranial end of the optic canal

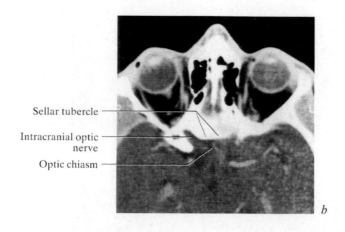

Sellar tubercle

Intracranial optic nerve

Optic chiasm

b

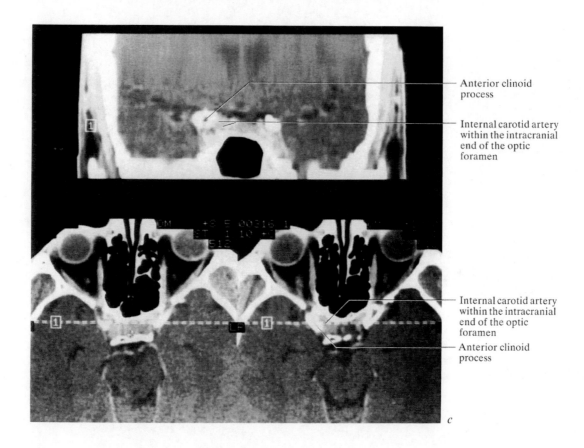

Anterior clinoid process

Internal carotid artery within the intracranial end of the optic foramen

Internal carotid artery within the intracranial end of the optic foramen

Anterior clinoid process

c

Fig. 70b, c

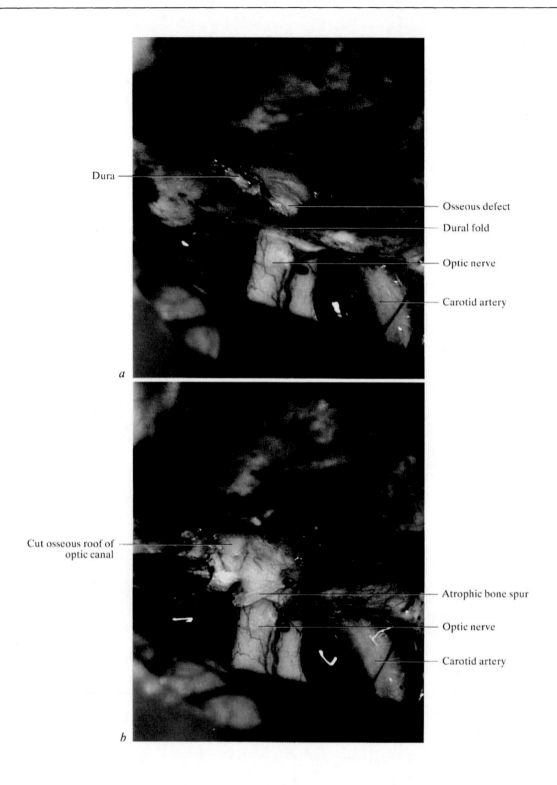

Dura —

— Osseous defect

— Dural fold

— Optic nerve

— Carotid artery

a

Cut osseous roof of — optic canal

— Atrophic bone spur

— Optic nerve

— Carotid artery

b

Fig. 71. (*a*) Intracisternal portion of the right optic nerve, the dura over the roof of the optic canal has been partially detached displaying an elliptic osseous defect of the roof. (Case 3 of selected reports.) (*b*) Following complete dissection of the dural fold covering the optic nerve an atrophic bone spur is removed

104

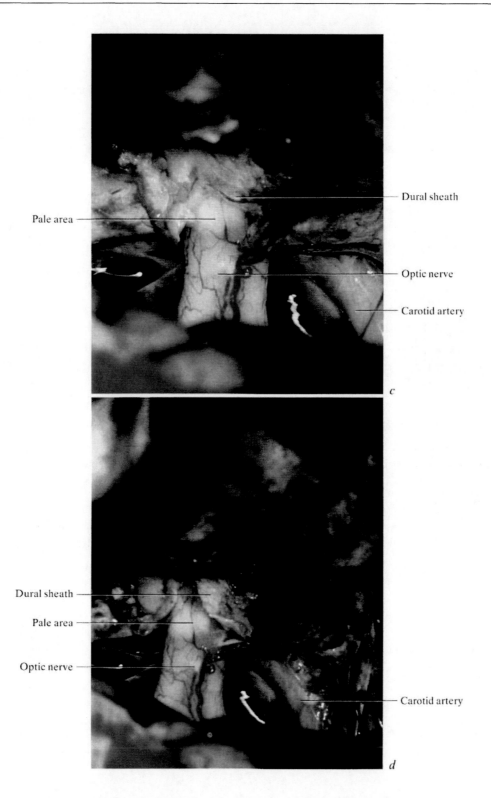

Fig. 71. (c) After partial opening of the dural sheath (DS) of the intracanalicular optic nerve (ON) a pale area (PA) with narrowed superficial vessels is observed underneath the elliptic osseous defect. (d) Complete opening of the dural sheath, the most distal portion of the optic nerve is not visualized. Superficial vessels narrowed within the area of the pale spot gain normal width beyond the lesion

105

Optic nerve compression by a dolichoectatic internal carotid artery causing visual loss and papilledema

A 66-year-old female reported at her first ophthalmological examination in September 1986 a roughly one-week history of blurred vision, a two-day history of darkness in front of her left eye and headaches which she projected in her forehead. There was a marked left afferent pupillary defect. Visual acuity in her right eye was 0.8, in her left eye 0.2. The right optic disk showed slight optic atrophy, the left chronic papilledema of about three diopters with beginning optic atrophy. Thin section CT was performed and revealed an enlargement of the cavernous sinus, dolichoectasia of the internal carotid artery, which reached deep into the left optic canal. The chiasm was in a "prefixed" position close to the tuberculum sellae. Both optic nerves appeared slightly enlarged. Optic nerve compression at the optic foramen was suspected and the patient underwent decompressive surgery by a pterional approach on October 6, 1986. At surgery the left optic nerve appeared flattened and pressed against the dural fold overcrossing the intracranial end of the optic canal. The postoperative course was complicated by thrombosis of the deep veins of the leg and a subdural hematoma, probably representing a complication of heparin therapy. Both were able to be treated successfully. After surgery, visual acuity increased from 0.2 to 0.4, the visual field showed only slight improvement, if at all, but papilledema resolved within ten days of surgery.

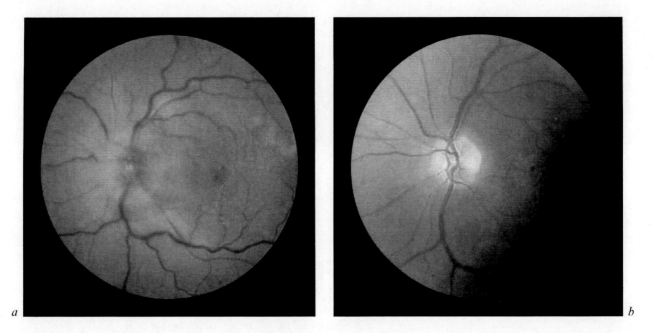

Fig. 72a, b. Photographs of the left optic disk before (*a*) and after (*b*) surgery. There is postoperative resolution of chronic papilledema leaving marked optic atrophy

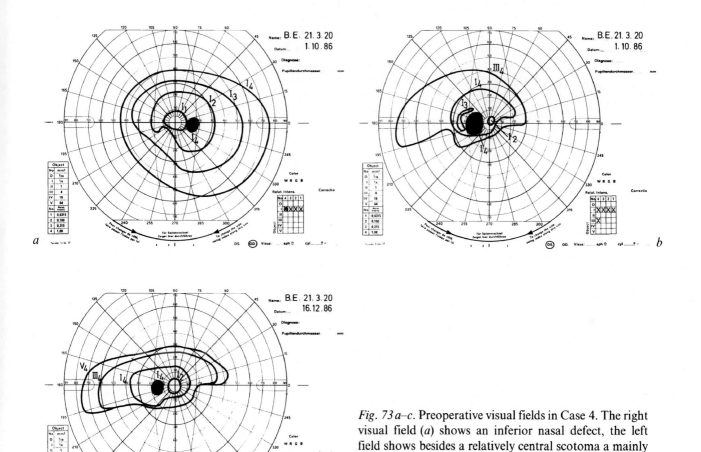

Fig. 73a–c. Preoperative visual fields in Case 4. The right visual field (*a*) shows an inferior nasal defect, the left field shows besides a relatively central scotoma a mainly inferior altitudinal defect with generalized constriction of the remaining upper half of the visual field (*b*). There is only slight improvement of the visual field after surgery (*c*)

107

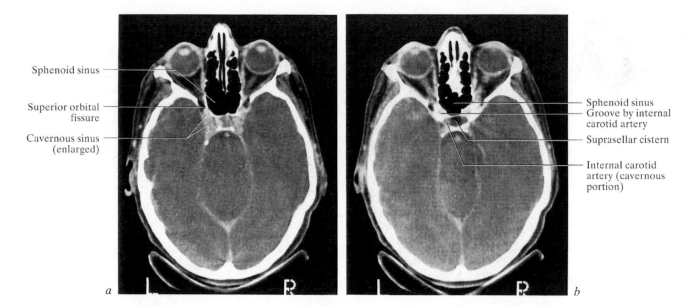

Sphenoid sinus

Superior orbital fissure

Cavernous sinus (enlarged)

Sphenoid sinus
Groove by internal carotid artery

Suprasellar cistern

Internal carotid artery (cavernous portion)

a

b

Fig. 74a–e. Axial anatomic CT sections in Case 4, (*a*) lowest, (*e*) highest section. The left cavernous sinus appears enlarged, probably due to dolichoectasia of the intracavernous portion of the internal carotid artery, the supraclinoid portion of which shows dolichoectasia. Both siphons of the internal carotid artery bulge into the neighboring sphenoid sinus and seem to elevate the floor of the optic canals (*b*), which appear narrowed (*c*). Part of the intracavernous portion of the enlarged artery on the left more than on the right side can be seen to extend into the suprasellar cistern (*b*). The left optic foramen is almost completely filled with dense soft tissue representing the supraclinoid portion of the artery (*c, d*). The almost cross-sectioned right internal carotid artery is visualized just at the intracranial opening of the right optic canal (*c*). The chiasm has an anterior and inferior "prefixed" position immediately next to the tuberculum sellae, indicating a short intracranial portion of the optic nerves (*e*)

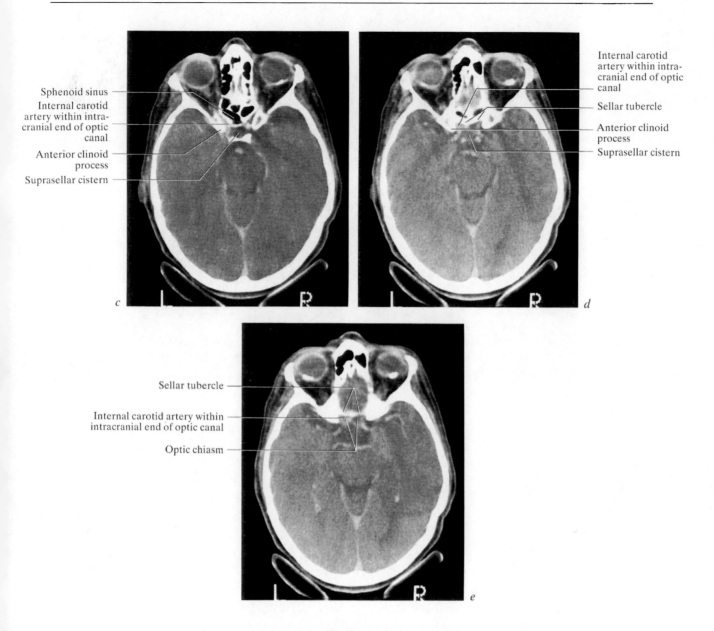

Sphenoid sinus

Internal carotid artery within intra-cranial end of optic canal

Anterior clinoid process

Suprasellar cistern

Internal carotid artery within intra-cranial end of optic canal

Sellar tubercle

Anterior clinoid process

Suprasellar cistern

Sellar tubercle

Internal carotid artery within intracranial end of optic canal

Optic chiasm

Fig. 74 c–e

109

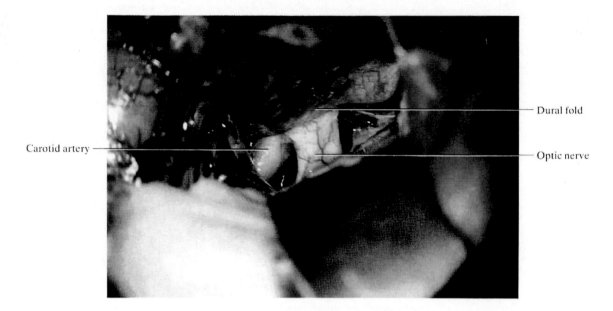

Carotid artery ─

─ Dural fold

─ Optic nerve

Fig. 75. Intraoperative findings in Case 4. The left optic nerve appears flattened and pressed against the dural fold overcrossing the intracranial end of the optic canal by the internal carotid artery

Summary

A 66-year-old female presented visual loss, an inferior altitudinal defect and chronic papilledema in her left eye. CT showed evidence for left optic nerve compression within the optic foramen by a dolichoectatic left carotid artery. This mechanism could be verified during surgery. There was slight improvement of visual function and immediate resolution of papilledema after surgery.

*Bilateral pneumosinus dilatans of the sphenoid sinus and
lesser wing of the sphenoid bone with narrowing
of both optic foramina*

A 43-year-old female had a five-year history of chronic papilledema and progressive optic atrophy and visual loss in her left
eye. CT and radiography of the optic foramina after Rhese were
reported to show "normal findings". When she was examined
in July 1982 she was almost blind in her left eye, visual acuity
being reduced to hand movements within a small residual island
of the left visual field. Visual acuity of the right eye was reduced
to 0.7–0.8 p and a relative paracentral scotoma in the upper
nasal and lower temporal field of vision as well as slighty defec-
tive color vision was noted. Ophthalmoscopy showed chronic
disk edema with severe optic atrophy, congestion of small vessels
and drusen-like hyalin bodies in the lower temporal half of the
disk (Fig. 59b). The right optic disk showed slight incipient papilledema. Thin section CT was performed and revealed massive
hyperpneumatization of the sphenoid sinus extending into both
anterior clinoid progresses causing severe narrowing of the optic
foramina more marked on the left than on the right side. The
diagnosis of optic nerve compression was made and decompressive surgery was performed by a right pterional approach in
order to unroof the optic canal and to exclude an intracanalicular optic nerve sheath meningeoma. During surgery the CT findings of extreme narrowing of the optic canal could be verified,
no extra- or intradurally situated meningeoma could be found.
After surgery there was an immediate improvement of visual
acuity in the right eye from 0.8 p to 1.2. The paracentral scotomas had disappeared and color vision was normal. The incipient
papilledema resolved within a few days. Visual function remained stable for the following $4^1/_2$ years.

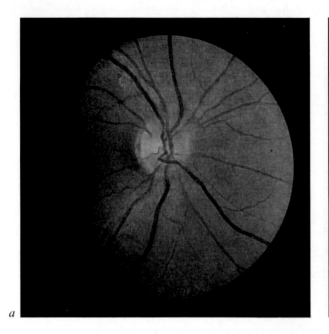
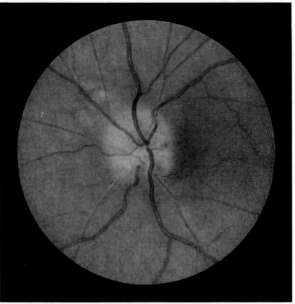

a

b

Fig. 76a, b. Fundus photographs of the optic disks in Case 5. There is incipient papilledema of the right (*a*) and chronic disk edema and severe optic atrophy of the left optic disk with congestion of small vessels and drusen-like hyalin bodies in the temporal lower quadrant of the left optic disk (*b*)

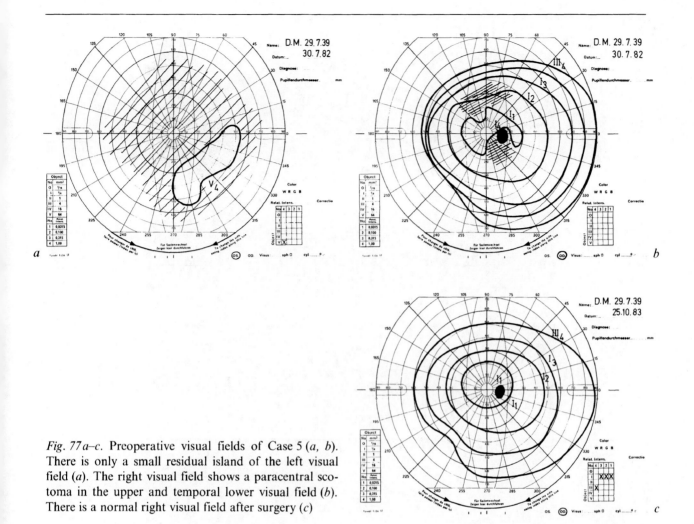

Fig. 77 a–c. Preoperative visual fields of Case 5 (a, b). There is only a small residual island of the left visual field (a). The right visual field shows a paracentral scotoma in the upper and temporal lower visual field (b). There is a normal right visual field after surgery (c)

113

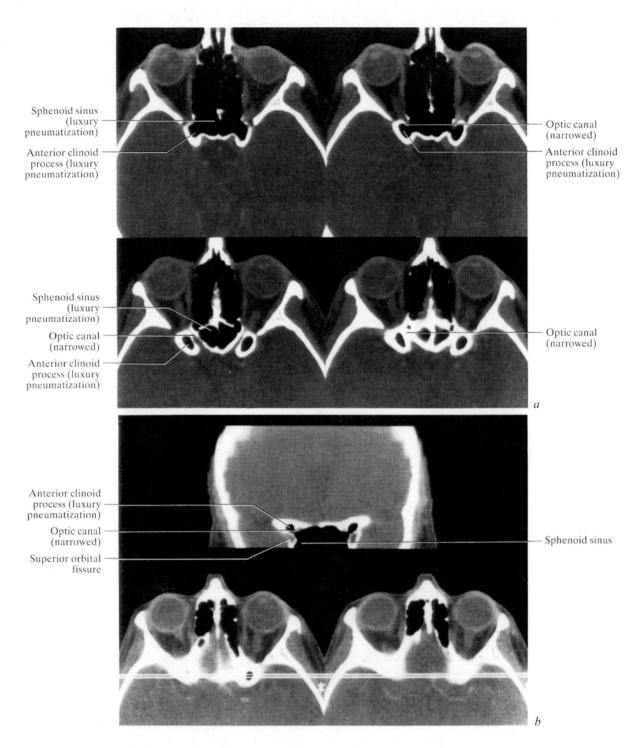

Sphenoid sinus
(luxury
pneumatization)

Anterior clinoid
process (luxury
pneumatization)

Optic canal
(narrowed)

Anterior clinoid
process (luxury
pneumatization)

Sphenoid sinus
(luxury
pneumatization)

Optic canal
(narrowed)

Anterior clinoid
process (luxury
pneumatization)

Optic canal
(narrowed)

a

Anterior clinoid
process (luxury
pneumatization)

Optic canal
(narrowed)

Superior orbital
fissure

Sphenoid sinus

b

Fig. 78. (a) Sequential axial anatomic sections (upper right lowest, lower left highest section) through both optic canals (bone window). There is considerable hyperpneumatization of the ethmoid and sphenoid sinuses, the latter extending continuously into the anterior clinoid processes resulting in marked narrowing of both optic canals. (b) Coronal computer reformation through the optic canals (above). The planum sphenoidale is elevated, the narrowed optic canals are visualized medially to the grossly pneumatized anterior clinoid processes. Pneumatization extends continuously from the sphenoid sinus into the anterior clinoid processes. The optic nerve shadows appear slightly enlarged, the left more marked than the right (below)

114

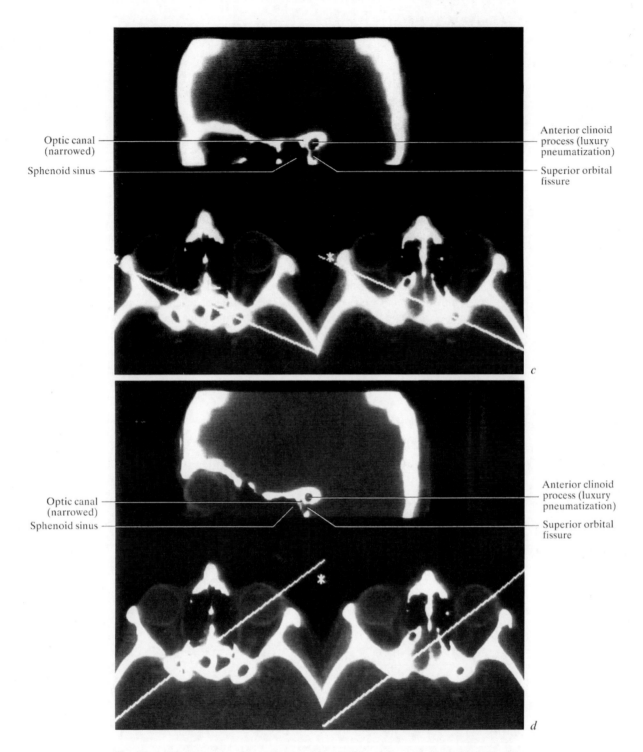

Optic canal (narrowed)

Sphenoid sinus

Anterior clinoid process (luxury pneumatization)

Superior orbital fissure

c

Optic canal (narrowed)

Sphenoid sinus

Anterior clinoid process (luxury pneumatization)

Superior orbital fissure

d

Fig. 78. (*c*) Computer reformation at about 90° to the course of the left optic canal comparable to the projection taken in conventional radiographs of the optic foramen after Rhese (above). The plane of section is indicated on the axial sections (below). The cross-sectioned pneumatized anterior clinoid process appears as a well defined roundish structure the size of a normal optic foramen, for which it can easily be mistaken. The optic canal proper is extremely narrowed and lies as a slit-like deformity medial to the anterior clinoid process. (*d*) Computer reformation at about 90° to the course of the right optic canal. The right optic foramen appears as a slit-like structure but is less narrowed than the left (*c*)

115

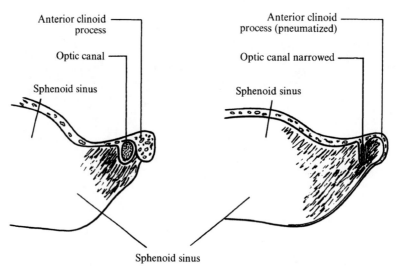

Anterior clinoid process

Optic canal

Sphenoid sinus

Anterior clinoid process (pneumatized)

Optic canal narrowed

Sphenoid sinus

Sphenoid sinus

Fig. 79. Schematic drawing of a slightly pneumatized but normal anterior clinoid process and optic canal (left) and the findings in case 5, where the optic canal is narrowed leading to optic nerve compression. (Same view as in Fig. 78c)

Summary

A 43-year-old woman with a history of progressive visual loss, chronic papilledema with optic atrophy leading to practical blindness of the left eye developed incipient papilledema and the clinical signs of right optic nerve compression. CT revealed a marked bilateral pneumosinus dilatans with narrowing of the optic canals. After decompressive surgery by a pterional approach visual function was immediately completely restored, incipient papilledema resolved and the finding remained stable for the following $4^1/_2$ years. No meningeoma was found extra- or intradurally.

Case 6 (K. G. 300940)

*Focal pneumosinus dilatans causing bone erosion and narrowing
of the left optic canal with optic nerve compression*

A 44-year-old male had his last ophthalmologic examination
in October 1983, when he suddenly dropped and fell on his head,
fracturing his skull, the trauma resulting in a left temporal contu-
sion. At that time he was found to have a visual acuity of 1.0
in both eyes and normal optic nerve heads. In June 1984 he
complained of fluctuating visual loss in his left eye with visual
acuity between 0.3 and 1.0. There was an insufficiently documented episode of slight left papilledema and retinal edema between the optic disk and the macula, probably due to a retinal
vascular occlusion. In May 1985 he experienced an acute episode
of visual loss from which he did not recover spontaneously.
At that time there was a marked afferent pupillary defect, color
vision was disturbed, and visual acuity had dropped to 0.32.
His left visual field showed besides a central scotoma a complete
inferior altitudinal defect and constriction of the remaining upper half of the visual field (Fig. 85a). Thin section CT was performed and revealed massive hyperpneumatization of the eth-
moidal air cells and sphenoid sinuses and a focal pneumatocele
which had eroded the lateral wall of the sphenoid sinus and
extended into the left optic canal, probably leading to optic
nerve compression. The patient underwent decompressive surgery, which verified focal ballooning of the sphenoid sinus into
the left optic canal, pressing the internal carotid artery and the
overlying optic nerve upward against the dural fold overcrossing
the optic foramen. Where the nerve was pressed against the
dural fold there was a deep rim within the nerve, the nerve
tissue being whitish and ischemic in this area. Proximal to the
rim there were numerous small new vessels, probably representing neovascularizations, and the arachnoid appeared locally
thickened. Immediately following surgery there was considerable
improvement of visual acuity and the patient was able to see
in the inferior half of the left visual field. On reexamination
about one week after surgery the patient's visual acuity had
increased from 0.32 to 1.0 and apart from the preexisting paracentral scotoma, which was probably due to a retinal vessel
occlusion, the visual field showed normal isopters (Fig. 85b).

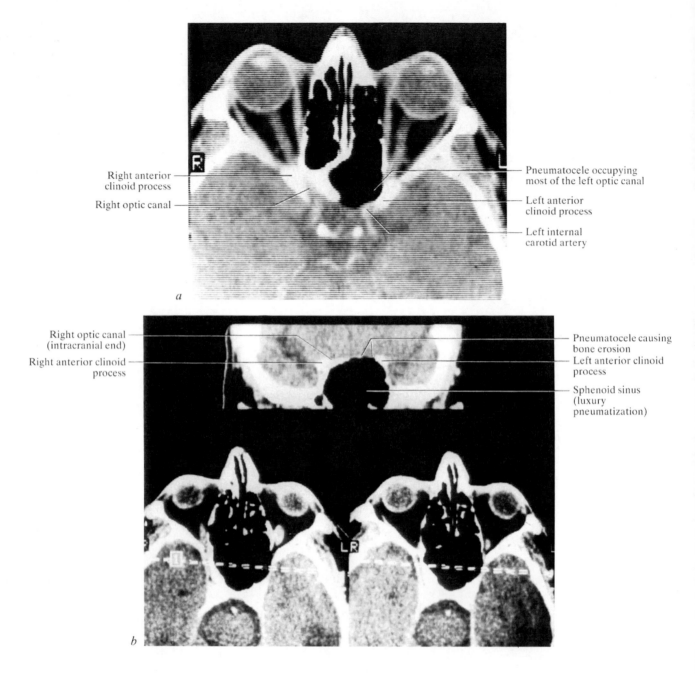

Right anterior clinoid process

Right optic canal

Pneumatocele occupying most of the left optic canal

Left anterior clinoid process

Left internal carotid artery

a

Right optic canal (intracranial end)

Right anterior clinoid process

Pneumatocele causing bone erosion

Left anterior clinoid process

Sphenoid sinus (luxury pneumatization)

b

Fig. 80 a, b

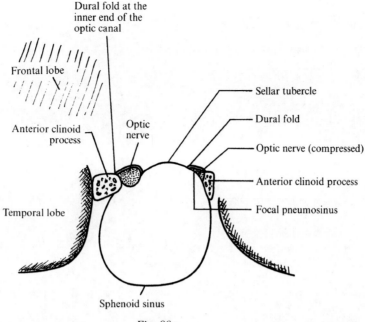

Fig. 80c

Fig. 80. (a) Axial CT section through both optic canals. There is a focal extension of the sphenoid sinus eroding the posterior lateral wall of the left sphenoid sinus reaching into the left optic foramen. The left internal carotid artery and left optic nerve are displaced. (b) Coronal computer reformation at the intracranial opening of the optic canal (above). Plane of section is indicated on the axial sections (below). Focal extension of the sphenoid sinus into the optic canal is well demonstrated. The sphenoid sinus is hyperpneumatized and ballooned. (c) Schematic drawing of the topography of Fig. 63b

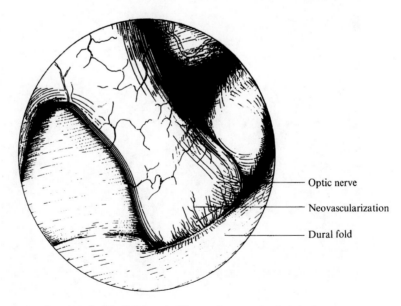

Fig. 81. Intraoperative sketch (Prof. Seeger). The optic nerve is slightly flattened and elevated by the internal carotid artery and pressed against the dural fold overcrossing the intracranial end of the optic foramen causing deep grooving. Proximal to the dural fold are numerous small vessels, probably representing neovascularizations

119

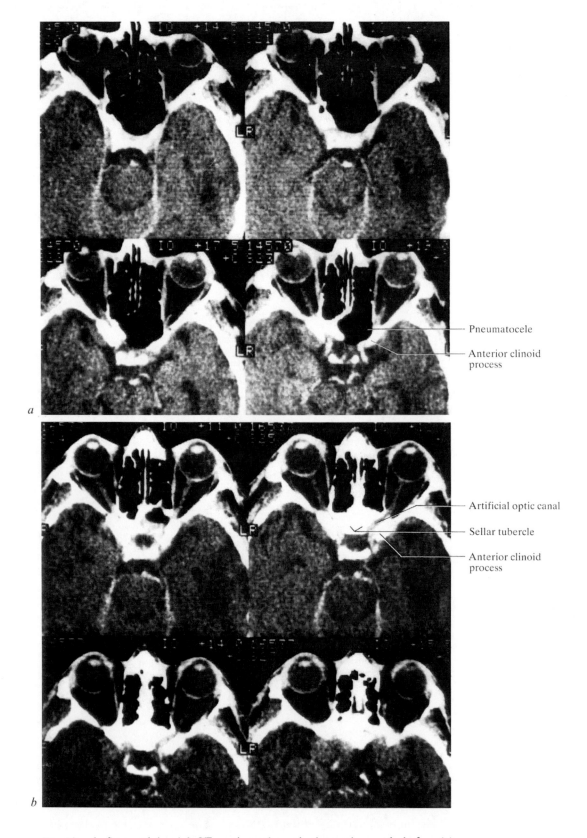

Pneumatocele

Anterior clinoid
process

Artificial optic canal

Sellar tubercle

Anterior clinoid
process

Fig. 82a, b. Sequential axial CT sections through the optic canals before (*a*)
and after (*b*) surgery. Surgical decompression by unroofing the optic canal has
created an artificial optic canal comparable to the topography of the unaffected
side

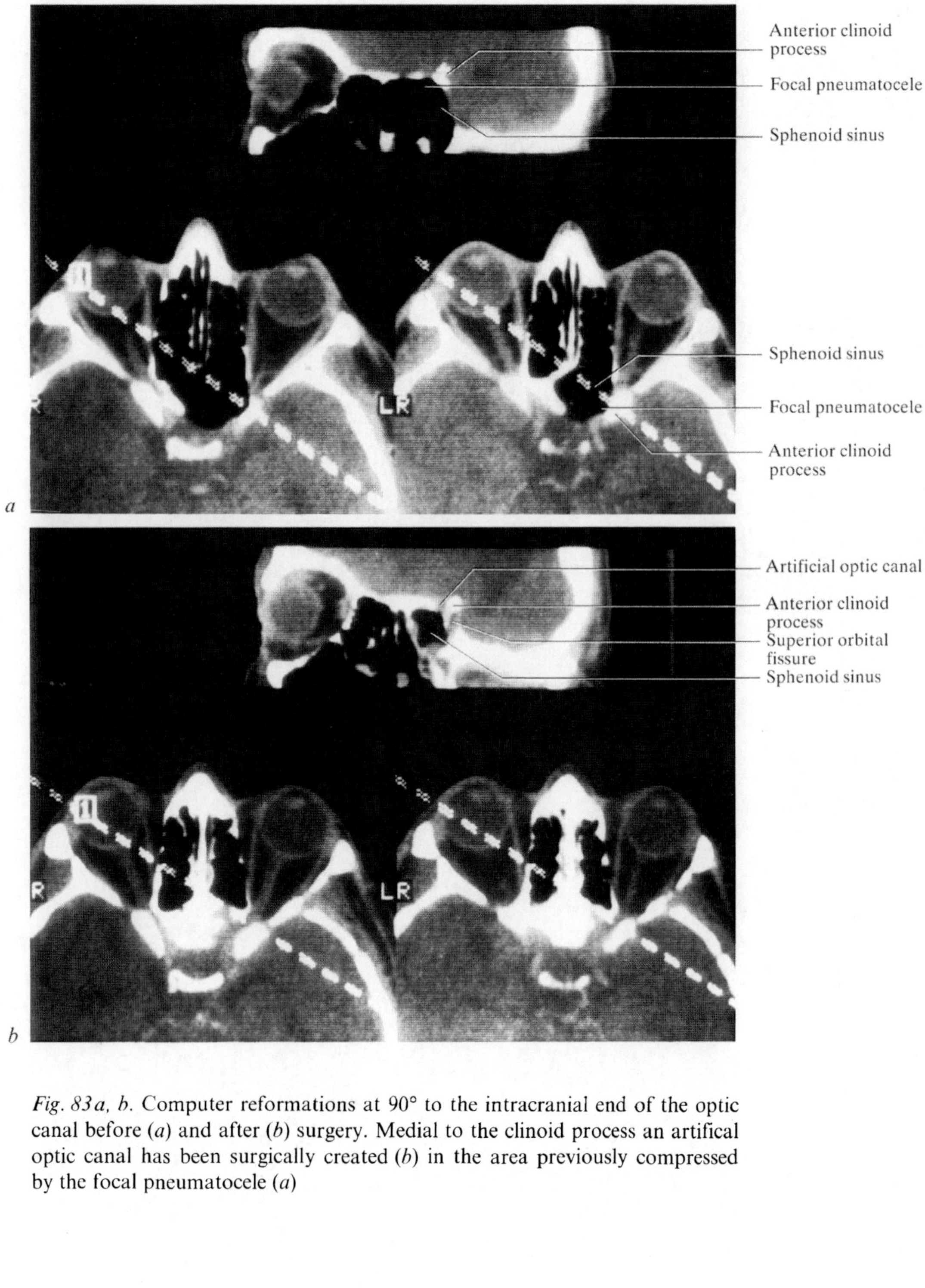

a
Anterior clinoid process
Focal pneumatocele
Sphenoid sinus
LR
Sphenoid sinus
Focal pneumatocele
Anterior clinoid process
b
Artificial optic canal
Anterior clinoid process
Superior orbital fissure
Sphenoid sinus
R
LR

Fig. 83a, b. Computer reformations at 90° to the intracranial end of the optic canal before (*a*) and after (*b*) surgery. Medial to the clinoid process an artifical optic canal has been surgically created (*b*) in the area previously compressed by the focal pneumatocele (*a*)

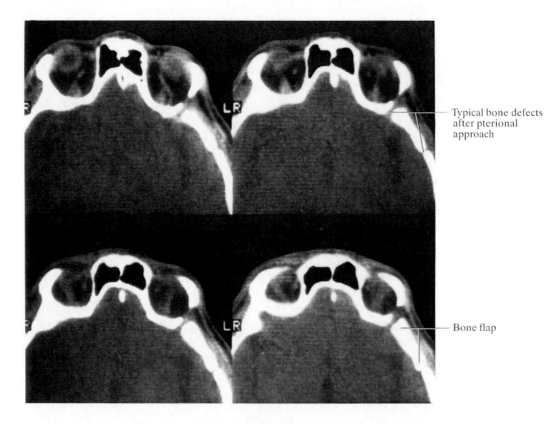

Typical bone defects after pterional approach

Bone flap

Fig. 84. Postoperative CT scan through the upper orbit (bone window) visualizing the characteristic bone defects after trepanation by a pterional approach

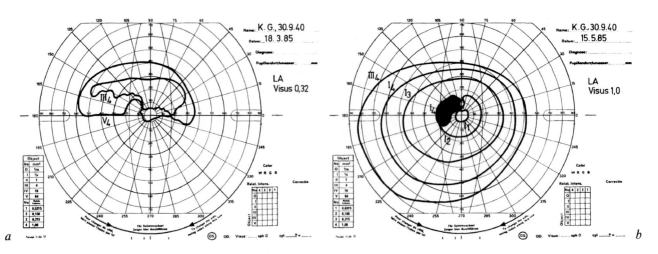

Fig. 85 a, b. Left visual field before (*a*) and after (*b*) surgery. Besides the central scotoma there is a complete inferior altitudinal defect and constriction of the remaining upper half of the visual field (*a*). After surgery the visual field is almost completely restored apart from a paracentral scotoma due to a previous retinal vascular occlusion

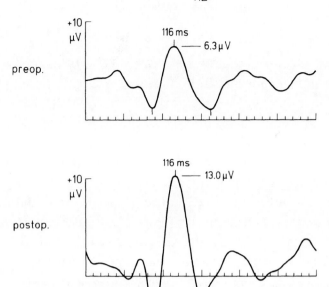

Fig. 86. Pre- and postoperative VEP of Case 6. There is considerable increase of the VEP amplitude reflecting the improvement of visual function (for details see Fig. 24a)

Summary

A 44-year-old male had intermittent episodes of visual loss in his left eye with fluctuating visual acuity between 0.3 and 1.0 for about 9 months. After another episode visual function did not recover spontaneously. Thin section CT showed a focal pneumosinus dilatans eroding the left optic canal and compressing the optic nerve. After decompressive surgery visual function returned almost completely.

*Optic nerve compression within a narrowed optic canal due
to focal hyperpneumatization (pneumosinus dilatans)*

A 36-year-old woman had observed progressive visual loss since
spring 1986. At the end of June she inadvertently covered her
left eye and realized that she was practically blind in her right
eye. At that time visual acuity in the right eye was reduced
to light perception in a small excentric island of the visual field.
There was a marked afferent pupillary defect and almost complete optic atrophy of the right disk, whereas the left disk appeared normal. Visual acuity in the right eye was after correction
of astigmatism 0.8, there was no significant visual field defect.
VEP of the left eye showed slight reduction of amplitude and
normal latency, possibly representing incipient blockage of nerve
conduction. Thin section CT showed very narrowed optic canals,
much more marked on the right than on the left side. On computer reformations through the optic canal a focal finger-like
extension of the sphenoid sinus was reaching into the midportion
of the optic foramen. The right optic nerve appeared slightly
thickened, probably due to chronic congestion or a small optic
nerve sheath meningeoma. The diagnosis of chronic optic nerve
compression was made and the patient underwent exploratory
surgery by a pterional approach mainly for exclusion of an intracranial extension of a possible optic nerve sheath meningeoma.
During surgery the optic canal was found to be narrow, the
optic nerve appeared atrophic and showed the characteristic
findings of local nerve compression. There was no evidence of
meningeoma. Postoperatively there was no change of visual
function, which had not been expected previously due to the
severe degree of optic atrophy.

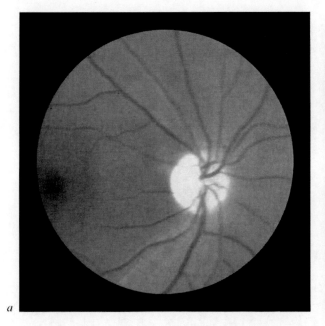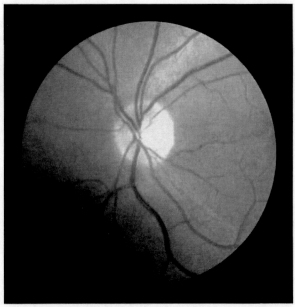

Fig. 87a, b. Fundus photographs of both optic disks in Case 7 prior to surgery. There is almost complete optic atrophy in the right eye (*a*) whereas the left optic disk appears normal

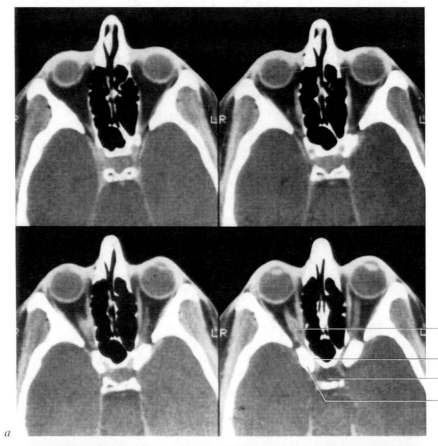

Optic nerve (orbital
portion) slightly
enlarged

Optic canal
(narrowed)

Suprasellar cistern

Anterior clinoid
process

a

b

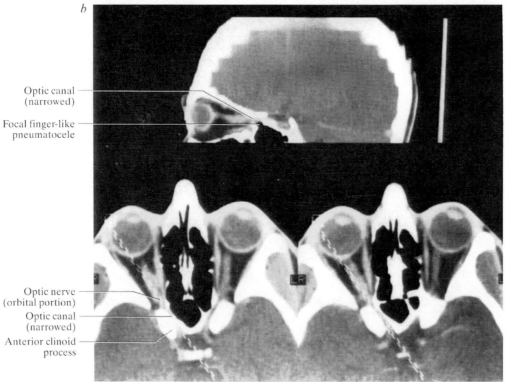

Optic canal
(narrowed)

Focal finger-like
pneumatocele

Optic nerve
(orbital portion)

Optic canal
(narrowed)

Anterior clinoid
process

◁ *Fig. 88.* (*a*) Sequential axial CT sections through the optic canals (upper right lowest, lower left, highest section): Both optic canals are very small, more marked on the left than on the right side. The right optic nerve is enlarged. (*b*) Computer reformation parallel to the course of the right optic canal (above). The plane of section is indicated on the axial CT sections (below). There is a focal finger-like extension of the sphenoid sinus into the right optic canal causing almost complete occlusion of the midportion of the right canal. The high density structure in front of the intracranial end of the optic foramen, partially obturating it, can be identified on the axial sections (below) as the right internal carotid artery

Summary

A 36-year-old female experienced progressive visual loss in her right eye with almost total optic atrophy without disk swelling. CT showed generalized and focal narrowing of the right optic canal due to a finger-like extension of the sphenoid sinus. Surgery revealed the signs of focal optic nerve compression but no meningeoma. Enlargement of the right optic nerve could represent a sign of chronic congestion (like in Case 5 with focal pneumosinus dilatans) but the presence of an orbital optic nerve sheath meningeoma can not be excluded with ultimate certainty. There was no postoperative improvement of visual function, but this could not possibly be expected with the high degree of preexisting optic atrophy.

10
Conclusions

The postoperative functional results presented in the case reports of this monograph seem to favor early microsurgical therapy of compressive lesions at the optic canal *before* optic atrophy has occurred. The precondition for *timely surgical intervention,* however, is an early diagnosis made jointly by the clinician and the radiologist. Both must be familiar with the signs pointing to optic nerve compression: the former with the clinical symptoms, the latter with the computed tomographic signs. Some of the disease entities responsible for optic nerve compression are ill-known to both. This applies particularly to pneumosinus dilatans and dolichoectatic vascular changes, the true incidence and natural course of which remain unclear. Familiarity with these lesions and appropriate CT examination techniques may in the future enable better estimation and optimal treatment of these conditions based on a larger sample of patients. Before such data are available, the indication for decompressive surgery should mainly be limited to those patients who show both the clinical signs and radiological findings that lead one to suspect optic nerve compression. Decompressive surgery should preferably be performed by experienced neurosurgical microsurgeons. Otherwise, the authors fear a "boom" of false positive diagnoses and therapeutic failures which could discredit the concept of these disease entities forever, leaving those patients who could profit from adequate therapy deprived of it.

References

Abelsdorff G (1928) In: Henke u. Lubarsch's Handbuch der speziellen pathologischen Anatomie und Histologie, Bd II. Springer, Berlin

Adson AW (1941) Surgical treatment of vascular diseases altering the function of the eyes. Trans Am Acad Ophthal Otolaryngol 46:95–111

Agati D (1940) Ipertrofie etmoido-sfenoidali a protrudenza endocrania. Radiol Med (Torino) 32:151–154

Agati D, Bertolotti M (1940) Protrusione endocrania di cellule etmoidosfenoidali con sindrome oculochiasmatica. Arch Radiol (Napoli) 31:16–24

Alpers BJ, Wolman IJ (1931) Arteriosclerotic disease of the optic nerve. Arch Ophthalmol 6:21–25

Anderson DR, Davis EB (1974) Retina and optic nerve after posterior ciliary artery occlusion. Arch Ophthalmol 92:422–426

Behr C (1911) Zur Entstehung der Optikusveränderungen bei Turmschädel. Ber Ophthalmol Ges Heidelberg 1910. Bergmann, Wiesbaden

Bendescu T (1932) Beiderseitige Optikusatrophie verursacht durch Pneumosinus dilatans der rechten Keilbeinhöhle. Z Augenheilkd 79:41–45

Benjamins CE (1918) Pneumosinus frontalis dilatans. Otolaryngol (Stockholm) 1:412–417

Bergaust B (1963) Unusual course of the internal carotid artery accompanied by bitemporal hemianopia. Acta Ophthalmol 41:270–274

Bernheimer S (1891) Über Sehnervenveränderungen bei hochgradiger Sklerose der Gehirnarterien. Graefes Arch Clin Exp Ophthalmol 37:37–57

Berson E, Freeman M, Gay A (1966) Visual field defects in giant suprasellar aneurisms of the internal carotid artery. Arch Ophthalmol 76:52–61

Beutel A, Tänzer A (1963) Röntgendiagnostik der Orbitae, der Augen und der Tränenwege. In: Handbuch der Med Radiologie, Bd VII/2. Springer, Heidelberg, S 683, 771ff

Boghen DR, Glaser JS (1975) Ischemic optic neuropathy. Brain 98:689–708

Bogousslavsky J, Steck AJ (1986) Bilateral third nerve palsy and anterior ischemic optic neuropathy. Neuroophthalmology 6:117–120

Brihaye J (1976) Neurosurgical approaches to orbital tumors. In: Krayenbühl H et al (eds) Advances and technical standards in neurosurgery. Springer, Wien New York, pp 103–121

Caramazza F (1932) Sindrome chiasmatica da ateromasia della carotide interna. Riv Otoneurooftalm 9:486–515

Cogan DG (1966) Neurology of the visual system. Thomas, Springfield

Cushing H (1930) The chiasmal syndrome of primary optic atrophy and bitemporal field defects in adults with an normal sella turcica. Arch Ophthalmol 5:505–733

Decker GR, et al. (1960) Klinische Neuroradiologie. Thieme, Stuttgart

De Schweinitz GE (1923) Concerning certain ocular aspects of pituitary body disorders, mainly exclusive of the usual central and peripheral hemianopie field defects. Trans Ophthalmol Soc UK 43:12–109

Diener HC, Zimmermann C (1985) Visual evoked potentials: recording problems and stimulation technique. EEG EMG 16:155

Dodd GB, Jing BS (1977) Radiology of the nose, paranasal sinuses and nasopharynx. Williams and Wilkins, Baltimore

Ellenberger C (1979) Ischemic optic neuropathy as a possible early complication of vascular hypertension. Am J Ophthalmol 88:1045–1051

Enoksson P (1965) Perimetry in neuro-ophthalmological diagnosis. Acta Ophthalmol [Suppl] (Copenh) 82:28–29

Enoksson P, Johannson JO (1978) Altitudinal field defects and retinal nerve fibre degeneration in optic nerve lesions. Acta Ophthalmol 56:957–968

Feldmann (1923) Pneumosinus et pneumatocèle. J Russe de nez, de la gorge et des oreilles 4:696–700

Fleischer K (1966) Zur Entstehung und Behandlung der Stirnhöhlenpneumocele. Arch Ohr Nas Kehlk-Heilkd 185:737–742

François J (1947) L'Hémianopsie binasale. Ophthalmologica 113:321–328

Fuchs E (1922) Senile changes of the optic nerve. Am J Ophthalmol 5:215–218

Fujioka M, Young LW (1978) The sphenoidal sinuses: Radiographic patterns of normal development and abnormal findings in infants and children. Radiology 129:133–136

Fukado Y (1975) Results in 400 cases of surgical decompression of the optic nerve. Mod Probl Ophthalmol 14:474–481

Glees M (1938) Dem Foster Kennedy'schen Syndrom ähnliche Veränderungen der Sehnerven durch Arteriosklerose. Klin Monatsbl Augenheilkd 100:865–873

Graefe A von (1857) Über die Iridektomie bei Glaucom und über den glaucomatösen Prozess. Graefes Arch Clin Exp Ophthalmol 3:456–555

Güttner HG (1942) Formbeeinflussung der Nebenhöhlen des Schädels durch vorzeitige Nahtsklerose. Beitr Path Anat 107:271–299

Gutman I, Behrens M, Odel J (1984) Bilateral central and centrocoecal scotomata due to mass lesions. Br J Ophthalmol 68:336–342

Hajek M (1926) Zwei verschiedene, bisher nicht beschriebene Tumorarten der Stirnhöhle und des Siebbeinlabyrinthes in ein und demselben Individuum. Passow-Schäfers Beitr 23:465–510

Halliday AM (1976) Visually evoked responses in optic nerve disease. Trans Ophthalmol Soc UK 96:372–376

Halliday AM, Halliday E, Kriss A, McDonald WI, Mushin J (1976) The pattern-evoked potential in compression of the anterior visual pathways. Brain 99:357–374

Hamby WB (1964) Pterional approach to the orbits for decompression or tumor removal. J Neurosurg 21:15–18

Harms H (1958) Augenheilkunde in Klinik und Praxis. In: Rohrschneider W (Hrsg) Fortbildungskurs für Augenärzte. München 1957. Enke, Stuttgart

Harms H (1962) Leitsymptom „Zentralskotom". Entwicklung und Fortschritt in der Augenheilkunde. Enke, Stuttgart

Hart WM, Burde RM, Klingele TG, Perlmutter JC (1980) Bilateral optic nerve meningeomas. Arch Ophthalmol 98:149–151

Hassler W, Eggert HR (1985) Extradural and intradural microsurgical approaches to lesions of the optic canal and the superior orbital fissure. Acta Neurochir (Wien) 74:87–93

Harz WM, Burde RM, Klingele TG, Perlmutter JC (1980) Bilateral optic nerve meningeomas. Arch Ophthalmol 98:149–151

Hayreh SS (1975) Anterior Ischemic optic neuropathy. Springer, New York

Hayreh SS (1981) Posterior ischemic optic. Neuropathy 182:29–41

Hayreh SS, Podhajski P (1979) Visual field defects in anterior ischemic optic neuropathy. Doc Ophthalmol 19:53–71

Henschen SE (1911) Über circumscripte arterosclerotische Nekrosen (Erweichungen) in den Sehnerven, im Chiasma und im Tractus. Graefes Arch Clin Exp Ophthalmol 78:212–223

Hippel EV (1923) Die Krankheiten des Sehnerven. In: Axenfeld u. Elschnig's Handbuch der gesamten Augenheilkunde. Springer, Berlin

Hirst LW, Miller NR, Allen GS (1979) Sphenoidal pneumosinus dilatans with bilateral optic nerve meningiomas. J Neurosurg 51:402–407

Hirst LW, Miller NR, Hodges FJ, Corbett JJ, Thompson S (1982) Sphenoid pneumosinus dilatans. A sign of meningioma originating in the optic canal. Neuroradiology 22:207–210

Hollenhorst RW, Hollenhorst RW Sr, MacCarty CS (1978) Visual prognosis of optic nerve sheath meningeomas producing shunt vessels on the optic disc. Mayo Clin Proc 53:84–92

Horniker (1924) Bericht der Deutschen Ophthalmologischen Gesellschaft, p 283

Housepian EM (1978) Microsurgical anatomy of the orbital apex and principles of transcranial orbital exploration. Clin Neurosurg 25:556–573

Hoyt WF (1962) Anatomic consideration of arcuate scotomas associated with lesions of the optic nerve and chiasm. A nauta axon degeneration study in the monkey. Bulletin of the John Hopkins Hospital, vol III, no 2, pp 57–71

Huber A (1971) Eye symptoms in brain tumors, 2nd edn. Mosby, St Louis, pp 221–225

Imachi J (1967) Neuro-surgical treatment of Lebers optic atrophy and its pathogenetic relationship to arachnoiditis. In: Progress in ophthalmology, vol 2. Preceedings of the Second International congress of Neurogenetics and Neuroophthalmology. Excerpta, Montreal, pp 121–127

Jain KK (1970) Saccular Aneurism of the ophthalmic artery. Am J Ophthalmol 69:997–998

Jefferson G (1937) Compression of the chiasma, optic nerves and optic tracts by intracranial aneurisms. Brain 60:444–497

Jezegabel C (1960) Manifestations oculaires du pneumosinus dilatans. Arch Ophthalmol 20:28–47

John ER (1973) Brain evoked potentials: Acquisition and analysis. In: Thomson RF, Patterson MM (eds) Bioelectric recording techniques. Academic Press, New York

Kahler O (1950) Zur Frage der Entstehung des Pneumatocelen der Stirnhöhle. Z Laryngol Rhinol 29:363–370

Kaufman B, Nulsen FE, Weiss MH et al (1977) Acquired spontaneous, nontraumatic normal pressure cerebrospinal fluid fistulas originating from the middle fossa. Radiology 122:379–387

Kaufman DI, Wray SH, Lorance R, et al (1986) An analysis of the pathophysiology and the development of treatment strategies for compressive optic nerve lesions using pattern electroretinogram and visual evoked potential. Neurology [Suppl 1] 36:232

Kearn TP, Rucker CW (1958) Arcuate defects in the visual fields due to chromophobe adenoma of the pituitary gland. Am J Ophthalmol 45:505–507

Kennedy F (1911) Retrobulbar neuritis as an exact diagnosis sign of certain tumors and abscesses in the frontal lobes. Am J Med Sci 141:355

Kennerdell JS, Maroon JC (1975) Intracanalicular meningioma with chronic optic disc edema. Am Ophthalmol 7:507–512

Kennerdell JS, Amsbangle GA, Myers EN (1976) Transantral-ethmoidal decompression of an optic canal fracture. Arch Ophthalmol 94:1040–1043

Killian H (1939) Pneumatopathien. Enke, Stuttgart, S 29

Klieneberger O (1913) Optikus Atrophie bei Gehirnarteriosklerose. Monatsschr Psychiatry Neurol 33:519–523

Knapp A (1932) On the association of sclerosis of the cerebral basal vessels with optic atrophy and cupping. Report of 10 cases. Trans Ophthalmol Soc UK 30:343–358

Knapp A (1940) Course in certain cases of atrophy of the optic nerve with cupping and low tension. Arch Ophthalmol 23:41–47

Knapp H (1875) Jahresbericht für Ophthalmologen, S 372

Koch I (1930) Kritisches Übersichtsreferat über die normale und pathologische Pneumatisation der Nebenhöhlen der Nase. Arch Ohr Nas Kehlk-Heilkd 125:174–218

Kupersmith MJ, Krohn D (1984) Cupping of the optic disc with compressive lesions of the anterior visual pathway. Ann Ophthalmol 16:948–953

Lang J (1981) Klinische Anatomie des Kopfes. Springer, Berlin Heidelberg New York

Lawwil T (1984) The bar pattern electroretinogram. Doc Ophthalmol 40:1–10

Leicher H (1928) Die Vererbung anatomischer Varianten der Nase, ihrer Nebenhöhlen und des Gehörganges. Bergman, München

Leonardi M, Fabris G (1976) Le pneumosinus dilatans, signe radiologique direct des mèningiomes de L'angle antérieur du chiasma. Am Radiologie 19:803–806

Ley A (1950) Compression of the optic nerve by a fusiform aneurism of the carotid artery. J Neurol Neurosurg Psychiatry 13:75–80

Liebrecht K (1902) Sehnerv und Arteriosklerose. Arch Augenheilkd 44:193–225

Lindenberg R, Walsh FB, Sacks JG (1973) Neuropathology of vision. Lea and Febiger, Philadelphia, pp 120, 174

Link R, Handl K (1954) Arch Ohr Nas Kehlk-Heilkd 165:403

Lisch W (1976) Doppelseitiges symetrisches Karotisaneurysma. Klin Monatsbl Augenheilkd 169:613–617

Lloyd GAS (1975) Radiology of the orbit. Saunders, London, pp 160–163

Lombardi G (1967) Radiology in neuro-ophthalmology. Williams and Wilkins, Baltimore, pp 163–166

Lombardi G, Passerini A, Cecchini A (1968) Pneumosinus dilatans. Acta Radiologica (Diagn) 7:535–542

Macialowicz T (1969) A case of dilating pneumosinus of the sphenoid sinus and posterior ethmoid cells. Polish Review of Radiol and Nuclear Med 23:324–330

Maffei L, Fiorentini A (1981) Electroretinographic responses to alternating gratings before and after section of the optic nerve. Science 211:953–954

Marchesani O (1937) Differentialdiagnostische Überlegungen bei Erkrankungen der vorderen Schädelgrube. Klin Monatsbl Augenheilkd 98:819–912

Matsuo K, Kobayashi S, Sugita K (1980) Bitemporal hemianopsia associated with sclerosis of the intracranial internal carotid arteries. Case report. J Neurosurg 53:566–569

Matsusaki H (1986) An experimental study on indirect injuries of the intracanalicular portion of the optic nerve. Neuroophthalmology 6:23–28

Mayer EG (1959) Diagnose und Differentialdiagnose in der Schädelröntgenologie. Springer, Wien

Mazzatesta F (1925) Lesioni endocraniele del nervo optico per arterosomia della caroticle e dell'oftalmica. Riv Otoneurooft 2:180–188

McCartney DL, Char DH (1985) Return of vision following orbital decompression after 36 hours of postoperative blindness. Am J Ophthalmol 100:602–604

McLean JM, Ray BS (1947) Soft glaucoma and calcification of the internal carotid arteries. Arch Ophthalmol 38:154–158

McLeod D, Marshall J, Kohner EM (1980) Role of axoplasmatic transport in the pathophysiology of ischemic disc swelling. Br J Ophthalmol 64:247–261

Meyer-Breiting E (1978) Spontaneous ethmoid pneumocele in chronic maxillary and ethmoid sinusitis and polyposis. HNO 26:350–352

Meyers AD, Burtschi T (1980) Pneumocele of the maxillary sinus. J Otolaryngol 9:361–363

Meyjes WP (1898) Mitteilung eines Falles vermutlicher Pneumatocele des Sinus frontalis. Monatsschr Ohrenheilkd 32:467–469

Michel J (1877) Über einige Erkrankungen des Sehnerven. Graefes Arch Clin Exp Ophthalmol 23:213–226

Miller NR (1982) In: Walsh and Hoyt's Clinical Neuro-Ophthalmology, 4th edn, vol 1. Williams and Wilkins, Baltimore London, p 334

Miller NR (1982) In: Walsh and Hoyt's Clinical Neuro-Ophthalmology, 4th edn, vol 1, Chap 15. Williams and Wilkins, Baltimore, London, pp 249–253

Mitts MG, McQueen JD (1965) Visual loss associated with fusiform enlargement of the intracranial portion of the internal carotid artery. J Neurosurg 23:33–37

Montresor D (1954) Esoftalmo unilaterale da cellula etmoidale ectopica simulante un tumore orbitario. Otoneurooftal (Bologna) 29:519–531

Morrison MD, Tchang SP, Maber RR (1976) Pneumocele of the maxillary sinus. Arch Otolaryngol 102:306–307

Morton ME (1983) Exzessive pneumatization of the sphenoid sinus. A case report. J Maxillofac Surg 11:236–238

Niho S, Niho M, Niho K (1970) Decompression of the optic canal by the transethmoidal route and decompression of the supraorbital fissure. Can J Ophthalmol 5:22–40

Nötzel H (1949) Über den Einfluß des Gehirns auf die Form der benachbarten Nebenhöhlen des Schädels. Dtsch Z Nervenheilkd 160:126–136; 162:956–361

O'Connell IEA, Du Boulay EPGH (1973) Binasal hemianopia. J Neurol Neurosurg Psychiatry 36:697–709

Olivecrona H (1927) Die chirurgische Behandlung der Gehirntumoren. Springer, Berlin

Oltersdorf U (1953) Die wirksamen Faktoren der Celenbildung. Arch Ohr Nas Kehlk-Heilkd 163:473–481

Oltersdorf U (1954) Die Wachstumskräfte und die formalen Vorgänge der normalen und pathologischen Pneumatisation des Gesichtsschädels. Habil Schrift, Tübingen

Otto R (1901) Sehnervenveränderungen bei Arteriosklerose und Lues. Arch Augenheilkd 43:104–124

Pages (1935) Les manifestations oculaires du Pneumosinus dilatans. Thèse, Lyon

Parin P (1951) Optikusatrophie durch Arteriosklerose der Carotis interna. Schweiz Arch Neurol Psychiatry 67:139–174

Persson HE, Wanger P (1984) Pattern-reversal electroretinograms and visual evoked cortical potentials in multiple sclerosis. Br J Ophthalmol 68:760–764

Petereit MF (1975) Orbital pseudoeffect secondary to excessive pneumatization of the sphenoid bone. SD J Med 28:5–7

Pfingst AO (1936) Anomalous ophthalmic artery with ocular symtoms. Arch Ophthalmol 16:829–838

Pincherle (1921) Über die röntgenographische Darstellung verkalkter Hirnarterien. Fortschr Geb Röntgenstr 29:215

Prott W (1977) Pneumosinus dilatans der Stirnhöhlen. Laryngol Rhinol Otol (Stuttg) 56:277–282

Psenner L (1963) Die Röntgendiagnostik der Nase, der Nasennebenhöhlen und des Epipharynx. In: Handbuch der Med Radiologie, Bd VII/2. Springer, Heidelberg

Püschel L, Schlosshauer B (1955) Über den Einfluß des somatotropen und androgenen Hormons auf die Pneumatisation. Arch Ohr Nas Kehlk-Heilkd 167:595–601

Quigley H, Anderson DR (1977) Cupping of the optic disc in ischemic optic neuropathy. Trans Am Acad Ophthalmol Otolaryngol 83:755–762

Quigley HA, Miller NR, Green WR (1985) The pattern of optic nerve fiber loss in anterior ischemic optic neuropathy. Am J Ophthalmol 100:769–776

Reicher MA, Bentson JR, Van Halbach V, et al (1986) Pneumosinus dilatans of the sphenoid sinus. AJNR 7:865–868

Repka MX, Savino PJ, Schatz NJ, et al (1983) Clinical profile and long-term implications of anterior ischemic optic neuropathy. Am J Ophthalmol 96:478–483

Ricci A, Werner A (1957) Vérification neurochirurgical du rôle des carotides internes dans certains symptoms chiasmatiques. Schweiz Med Wochenschr 87:1190–1198

Riggs LA, Johnson EP, Schick AML (1964) Electrical responses of the human eye to moving stimulus patterns. Science 144:567

Rönne (1924) Die klinischen Symptome der arteriosklerotischen Opticusatrophie. Acta Ophthalmol 2:160–166

Röpke F (1905) Verletzungen der Nase und deren Nebenhöhlen. Bergman, München, S 107

Röver J, Bach M (1987) The pattern ERG and the VEP in malingering patients. Doc Ophthalmol (in press)

Röver J, Bach M, Mack M, Oschwald M (1983) Die visuell evozierten Potentiale (VEP) bei Erkrankungen der Sehbahn. Fortschr Ophthalmol 79:506–508

Sacks JG, Lindenberg R (1969) Symptomatology and pathogenesis of arterial elongation and distension. The John Hopkins Medical Jour 125:95–106

Sandford HS, Craig W, Wagener HP (1936) An unusual chiasmal lesion and its operative treatment. Proc Staff-Meetings, Mayo-Clinic 10:721–730

Saphir O (1933) Changes of the optic nerve resulting from pressure of arteriosclerotic internal carotid arteries. Am J Ophthalmol 16:110–118

Sattler CH (1920) In: von Graefe A, Saemisch ET (Hrsg) Handbuch der gesamten Augenheilkunde, vol 1. Engelmann, Leipzig, S 2, 9

Schaeffer JP (1925) Some points in the regional anatomy of the optic pathway with especial reference to tumors of the hypophysis cerebri and resulting ocular changes. Anat Rec 28:243–279

Schiffer HK (1951) Cerebrale Frühschädigung und Schädeldysplasie. Fortschr Röntgenstr 75:54–59

Schildwächter A, Unsöld R (1987) Flüchtige Paresen bei Tumoren (transient cranial nerve palsies in compressive lesions). Z Prakt Augenheilkd 8:281–285

Schlezinger NS, Thompson RA (1967) Pituitary tumors with central scotomas simulating retrobulbar neuritis. Neurology 17:782–788

Schloffer H (1934) Erwägungen über die operative Entlastung des intrakraniellen Optikusabschnittes. Zugleich ein Beitrag zum Foster-Kennedyschen Syndrom. Med Klin 30:421–425

Schlosshauer B (1956) Die Beziehungen des Pneumosinus frontalis dilatans zur Stirnbeinpneumatisation. HNO 6:112–115

Schmidt D, Bührmann K (1977) Inferior hemianopia in parasellar and pituitary tumors. In: Glaser JS (ed) Neuro-ophthalmology, vol IX. Mosby, St Louis, pp 236–247

Schmidt R (1953) Über zwei seltene Druckschädigungen des Sehnerven. Klin Monatsbl Augenheilkd 123:546–552

Schüller A (1930) Über eine eigenartige Anomalie (Pneumocele des Sphenoids bei Tumoren der Hirnbasis). Monatsschr Ohrenheilkd 64:924–928

Schürmann K, Oppel O (1961) Die transfrontale Orbitotomie als Operationsmethode bei retrobulbären Tumoren. Klin Monatsbl Augenheilkd 139:129–259

Seeger W (1980) Microsurgery of the brain. Anatomical and technical principles (in two volumes). Springer, Wien New York

Seeger W (1983) Microsurgery of the cranial base. Springer, Wien New York

Seeger W (1986) Planning strategies of intracranial microsurgery. Springer, Wien New York

Selz BE (1970) Hyperpneumatisation der Keilbeinhöhe. Med Diss, Basel

Shearer DE, Dustman RE (1980) The pattern reversal evoked potential: the need for laboratory norms. Am J EEG Technol 20:185–200

Shearer DE, Creel D, Dustman RE (1983) Efficacy of evoked potential stimulus parameters in the detection of visual system pathology. Am J EEG Technol 23:137–146

Sofermann RA (1981) Sphenoethmoidal approach to the optic nerve. Laryngoscope 41:184–196

Sokol S, Moskowitz A (1981) Effect of retinal blur on the peak latency of the pattern evoked potential. Vision Res 21:1279–1286

Som PM, Sachden VP, Biller HF (1983) Sphenoid sinus pneumocele, report of a case. Arch Otolaryngol 109:761–764

Spoor TC, Mathog RH (1986) Restoration of vision after optic canal decompression. Arch Ophthalmol 104:804–806

Spoor TC, Kennerdell JS, Maroon JC (1981) Pneumosinus dilatans, Klippel-Trenaunay-Weber-Syndrome and progressive visual loss. Ann Ophthalmol 13:105–108

Stanka R (1933) Über Pneumosinus sphenoidalis und Optikusatrophie. Med Klin 29:980–981

Süsse HJ (1964) Das Pneumatisationsproblem der Stirnhöhlen in dynamischer Sicht. Arch Ohr Nas Kehlk-Heilkd 184:115–128

Sugita K, Sato O, Hirota T et al (1975) Scotomatous defects in the central visual field in pituitary adenomas. Neurochirurgia (Stuttg) 18:155–162

Sugita K, Hirota T, Iguchi I et al (1977) Transient amaurosis under decreased atmospheric pressure with sphenoidal sinus dysplasia. Case report. J Neurosurg 46:111–114

Susac JO, Martius AN, Whaley RA (1977) Intracanalicular meningioma with normal tomography. J Neurosurg 46:659–662

Tassman IS (1944) Foster Kennedy Syndrome with fusiform aneurism of internal carotid arteries. Arch Ophthalmol 32:125–127

Thiel R (1930) Glaucom ohne Hochdruck. 48. Verslg Ophthalmol Ges Heidelberg, S 133–136

Tomsak RL, Costin JA, Hanson M (1979) Carotid-ophthalmic artery aneurism presenting as unilateral disc edema with choroidal folds. In: Smith JL (ed) Neuroophthalmology Focus 1980. Masson, New York, pp 181–187

Torma T, Koskinen K (1961) A case of unilateral optic foramen meningioma. Acta Ophthalmol 39:460–465

Trobe J, Glaser JS, Cassady J, et al (1980) Nonglaucomatous excavation of the optic disc. Arch Ophthalmol 98:1046–1050

Türk L (1852) Über Compression und Ursprung des Sehnerven. Zeitschr Kais Kön Gesellsch der Ärzte Wien 8:299–304

Ungerecht K (1964) Der Pneumosinus frontalis dilatans. HNO 12:233–245

Unsöld R (1982) Zur computer-tomographischen Differentialdiagnose der Erkrankungen des Sehnerven. Graefes Arch Clin Exp Ophthalmol 219:124–138

Unsöld R (1983) Zur computer-tomographischen Diagnose von Läsionen der vorderen Sehbahn. Fortschr Ophthalmol 218:124–138

Unsöld R (1984) Sehnervenschäden durch Karotisdruck. Augenärztlicher Fortbildungsabend 07.12.84. Universitäts-Augenklinik Freiburg, Mitteilungen aus der Klinik 6/1984

Unsöld R (1987) Ophthalmologische Indikationen zur Computertomographie. Teil 1: Ophthalmoskopisch sichtbare Veränderungen, Visusminderung und Gesichtsfeldausfälle. Z Prakt Augenheilkd 8:21–28

Unsöld R, Degroot J, Newton TH (1980) Images of the optic nerve. Anatomic CT correlation. AJNR 1:317–323

Unsöld R, Newton TH, Hoyt WF (1980) CT-Examination technique of the optic nerve. J Comp Assist Tomogr 4:560–563

Unsöld R, Norman D, Berninger W (1980) Multiplanar evaluation of the optic canal from axial transverse CT sections. J Comp Assist Tomogr 4:418–419

Unsöld R, Ostertag CB, Degroot J, Newton TH (1982) Computer reformations of the brain and skull base. Anatomy and clinical application. Springer, Berlin Heidelberg New York

Vines FS, Bonstelle CT, Floyd HL (1976) Proptosis secondary to pneumocele of the maxillary sinus. Neuroradiology 11:57–59

Walsh FB (1957) Clinical neuro-ophthalmology, 2nd edn. Williams and Wilkins, Baltimore, p 33ff

Walsh FB (1971) Meningiomas primary within the orbit and optic canal. In: Smith JL (ed) Neuroophthalmology. Symposium of the University of Miami and the Bascom Palmer Eye Institute, vol 5, pp 240–266

Walsh FB, Hoyt WF (1969) Clinical neuro-ophthalmology, 3rd edn, vol 2. Williams and Wilkins, Baltimore, p 1774

Walsh FB, Hoyt WF (1969) In: Clinical neuroophthalmology, 3rd edn, vol 2, p 1748

Weickmann F (1958) Vikariierende Nebenhöhlenhyperplasie bei hypoplastischen Großhirnprozessen. Fortschr Röntgenstr 88:432–439

Wiggli U, Oberson R (1975) Pneumosinus dilatans and hyperpstosis. Early signs of meningeomas of the anterior chiasmatic angle. Neuroradiology 8:262–283

Wilbrand H, Saenger A (1913) Die Neurologie des Auges, Bd 5. Bergman, München

Williams JP, Shawker TH, Lora J (1975) Pneumosinus dilatans of the sphenoid sinus. Bull Los Angeles Neurol Soc 40:45–48

Wilson WB (1981) Meningiomas of the anterior visual system. Surv Ophthalmol 26:109–127

Wilson WB, Gordon M, Lehmann RAW (1979) Meningiomas confined to the optic canal and foramina. Surg Neurol 12:21–28

Wittmack K (1918) Über die normale und pathologische Pneumatisation des Schläfenbeins. Fischer, Jena

Wright JE, Call NK, Liaricoss S (1980) Primary optic nerve meningioma. Br J Ophthalmol 64:553–558

Wurster CF, Levine TM, Sisson GA (1986) Mucocele of the sphenoid sinus causing sudden onset of blindness. Otolaryngology-Head Neck Surg 94:257–259

Yasargil MG, Fox JL (1975) The microsurgical approach to intracranial aneurysms. Surg Neurol 3:7–14

Yaskin HE, Schlezinger NS (1942) Foster Kennedy Syndrome associated with non neoplastic intracranial conditions. Arch Ophthalmol 28:704–710

Yolton RL, Allen RG, Goodson RA, Schafer DL, Decker WD (1983) Amplitude variability of the steady-state visual evoked response (VER). Am J Optometry Physiol Optics 60:694–704

Yune HY, Holden RW, Smith JA (1975) Normal variations and lesions of the sphenoid sinus. Am J Roentgenol Radium Ther Nucl Med 124:129–138

Zanek J, Brihaye J (1948) L'hemianopsie horizontale opto-chiasmatique. Bull Sa Ophthal France, p 411

Zange J, Moser F (1940) Der Ductus nasofrontalis bei Stirnhöhlenerkrankungen und das Becksche Punktionsverfahren. Arch Ohr Nas Kehlk-Heilkd 147:114, 127

Zizmor J, Bryce M, Schaffer SL, Noyek AM (1975) Pneumocele of the maxillary sinus. Arch Otolaryngol 100:155–156

Zuckerkandl E (1893) Normale und pathologische Anatomie der Nasenhöhle und ihrer pneumatischen Anhänge. Braumüller, Wien Leipzig

Subject Index

Page numbers in *italics* refer to the principle discussion of subject

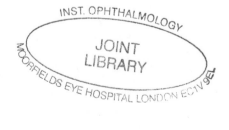
INST. OPHTHALMOLOGY
JOINT LIBRARY
MOORFIELDS EYE HOSPITAL LONDON EC1V 9EL

G. O. H. Naumann, University of Erlangen-Nürnberg;
D. J. Apple, University of Utah, Salt Lake City

Pathology of the Eye

With contributions by D. von Domarus, E. N. Hinzpeter,
R. M. Manthey, L. R. Naumann, K. W. Ruprecht, H. E. Völcker

Translated from the German by D. J. Apple

1986. 544 figures in 1002 parts. XXXV, 998 pages.
ISBN 3-540-96044-9

Contents: General Anatomy and Development of the Eye: Techniques of Investigation. – Microscopic Anatomy of the Eye. – Malformations and Anomalies of the Eye. – Intraocular Inflammations. – Accidental and Surgical Trauma and Wound Healing of the Eye. – Conjunctiva. – Cornea and Sclera. – Uvea. – Lens. – Vitreous. – Retina. – General Pathology of the Retina: Correlation of the Ophthalmoscopic Appearance with Tissue Morphology. – Optic Nerve. – Glaucoma and Ocular Hypotony: Pathology of Abnormal Intraocular Pressure. – Ocular Adnexae: Eyelids and Lacrimal Apparatus. – The Eye and Systemic Disease. – Morphology of Drug-Induced Ocular Changes. – Index.

From the foreword by F. C. Blodi
"This book represents a comprehensive, thorough and up-to-date clinical oriented textbook on ocular pathology.
…Nothing of this kind has so far been available in English. The book has a twofold purpose: First it is meant to be a source of instruction for ophthalmologists and pathologists. For that purpose it is beautifully illustrated both by clinical pictures and by excellent photomicrographs and electromicroscopic pictures. Most valuable from a didactic point of view are the colored schematic drawings and the many tables. These two features are practically unique and should help any neophyte in grasping the principles of ocular pathology.
The second objective of this book is as a reference book for any type of investigation concerned with ocular pathology. The list of references (exceeding 5,000 citations) is indeed staggering and reflects the thoroughness and scholarship of the authors. The references cover not only publications in German and English, but also many works published in other languages. This gives the book a true cosmopolitan character. **This book will become the yardstick against which any other future publications in ocular pathology will have to be measured.**"

Springer-Verlag Berlin
Heidelberg New York London
Paris Tokyo Hong Kong

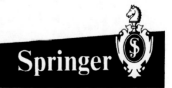

F. H. Stefani, G. Hasenfratz, University of Munich, Germany

Macroscopic Ocular Pathology

An Atlas Including Correlations with Standardized Echography

1987. 320 figures, mostly in color. XII, 178 pages.
ISBN 3-540-17404-4

Contents: Artifacts. – Cornea. – Sclera. – Uveal tract. – Retina and macula. – Vitreous. – Lens. – Optic nerve. – Glaucoma. – Tumors and pseudotumors. – Trauma. – Index.

This is a unique atlas presenting macroscopic ocular pathology with correlated ocular ultrasound. Its objective is not to cover every known pathological condition, but to include illustrations which may contribute to the understanding of clinical findings. Moreover, clinicians, practitioners, students and residents may need the macroscopic image of a diseased organ in order to correlate the technical findings of ultrasound, CT scanning, or scintigraphy with clinical conditions.

The chapters deal with the various ocular structures in sequence and address mainly malformations, inflammatory reactions, degenerative lesions and secondary tissue reactions, glaucoma, ocular trauma (both accidental and surgical), tumors, and socalled pseudotumors. Since intraocular microsurgery has become routine over the past decade, vitreo-retinal reactions have attracted more interest and are hence documented in greater detail.

This atlas will provide a supplement to existing texts and will stimulate clinical and diagnostic progress.

Springer-Verlag Berlin
Heidelberg New York London
Paris Tokyo Hong Kong

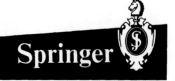

Springer

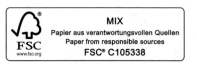

MIX
Papier aus verantwortungsvollen Quellen
Paper from responsible sources
FSC® C105338
FSC
www.fsc.org

Printed by Books on Demand, Germany